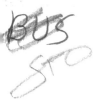

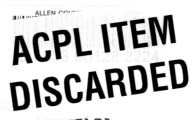

Y0-BST-853

7-12-76

THE
ONE-HANDER'S
BOOK

THE ONE-HANDER'S BOOK

A Basic Guide to Activities of Daily Living

VERONICA WASHAM

Photographs by Mark Feldstein

THE JOHN DAY COMPANY / AN INTEXT PUBLISHER

New York

Library of Congress Cataloging in Publication Data

Washam, Veronica.
    The one-hander's book.

    1. Physically handicapped. 2. Amputees. I. Title.
[DNLM: 1. Activities of daily living—pop. wks.
2. Amputees—popular works. 3. Arm—popular works.
4. Hand—popular works. 5. Rehabilitation—popular
works. HD7255 W314o 1973]
HV3011.W29   613   77-155019
ISBN 0-381-97096-5

The John Day Company, 257 Park Avenue South, New York, N.Y. 10010

Published on the same day in Canada by Longman Canada Limited.

Printed in the United States of America.

HANDICAP

"... a race or contest in which, in order to equalize chances of winning, an artificial disadvantage is imposed on a supposedly superior contestant...."

Webster

CONTENTS

AUTHOR'S NOTE

This guide is written primarily to benefit persons who have lost full or partial use of an arm through accident or injury, stroke, amputation, birth defect, or an illness such as polio. Included, of course, are returning servicemen with arm injuries. The techniques presented apply to everyone—to teenagers, adults, men, and women—but they will work best for persons having one well-functioning arm, hand, and five fingers, and good use of the legs and body. Acquired and proved by years of practical application, these techniques were developed by a right-hander but are equally adaptable to left-handed use. In special instances where adaptation is rather unusual, as for instance, for certain requirements of ballroom dancing, the author has tried to reconstruct the activity so that it will be acceptable.

INTRODUCTION

In the beginning it may seem difficult to cope with a permanent loss that necessitates the reorganization of one's life pattern. Recent one-handers may have a particularly hard time adjusting emotionally and psychologically to the idea of going through life with one arm. This feeling should not persist for long, however. Many people find that it can be ameliorated by seeking professional help to regain a proper perspective. It is perfectly normal for some also to experience a realistic anxiety arising from the realization that an accident or injury to the remaining good arm can impair one's ability to function, leaving one partially or totally dependent on others. In this connection the one-handed person may want to inquire into the feasibility of insurance coverage.

Admittedly, if you have grown up with one arm, adjusting is a great deal easier than if you find yourself with an arm just rendered useless or have had one amputated after you have reached adulthood. It will also be easier to adjust to one-handed living if the dominant arm remains the useful one. There is no pretending that learning to do everything with one hand will be easy, particularly if one has become one-handed after about the middle teens. But we hope to help even latecomers to master the techniques of living with one arm without having to ask for help or having to use special equipment or mechanical aids.

In this era of modern conveniences, with more coming along every year, being one-handed is much less a hardship than it must have been even a generation ago. Many of the time- and labor-saving implements devised for two-handed persons can be used by one-handers. However, this is not a book about gadgets or especially constructed devices. We assume that the one-handed person does not wish to be dependent on special aids or to stand out against an artificial background created of specialized equipment. We live in the two-hander's world and it is more practical and reasonable to adapt to it than to ask that world to adapt to us.

One-handers who still have the second, nonfunctioning, arm or an artificial one have an advantage, because this arm can be useful in several ways: as a weight for holding light materials steady; as the means, with the help of the good arm, of circling an object to be lifted or carried, such as a large package or even a child. Other uses for the secondary arm are found throughout the book. Putting the nonfunctioning arm to gentle use with intelligence and care cannot harm it in any way; rather it may serve to strengthen it, thus affording minimal function, which is all to the good. Those having an artificial arm can put it to much greater use with perhaps 50 percent greater efficiency. Your good arm by virtue of the double duty it performs will also become considerably stronger than it was previously. This is the natural law of physical compensation at work. Another way in which compensation manifests itself is that other parts of the body will take over some of the work of a lost or injured part. The parts that accommodate the one-hander most frequently are the knees, the midsection, the lap, and the feet.

One-handers need not be timid about approaching an untried task or situation, for they may trust their own judgment as to what and how much they can do, and should set their own pace and their own limitations. After all, life gives us as much or as little as we accept.

Sometimes well-meaning relatives and friends may be restrictive in their attitudes about what constitutes safety or nonsafety. It is natural for them to feel anxious and to express intelligent, pertinent fears about limitations and abilities. In such cases we recommend communicating to others exactly what you are able and prepared to perform without help. The direct approach is best—a simple statement such as "You are probably wondering how I manage to do such and such...."—then proceed to explain precisely how you accomplished the task in question. Thus, as you are letting others know how you would like to be treated, you shift attention from the physical to the inner self.

As your confidence increases you will be tackling activities usually regarded as being only for two-handers, such as piano playing. Depending on where your interests lie, you can learn, or relearn, the techniques for swimming, carpentry, sewing, driving a car, and others, and generally function as efficiently as your friends, neighbors, family, and co-workers. It may take you a little longer to perform such activities, particularly in the beginning, but with practice you will not be far behind. Your patience, effort, and determination will be rewarded by efficiency, renewed faith, and restored independence.

Most of all, keep your sense of humor alive! Try to enjoy the humorous incidents you may encounter as you reorient yourself to living with your one hand. Some situations can provoke either a chuckle or a frown. The chuckle will go a long way toward brightening your life. We who are one-handers must always remember that our attitude about ourselves largely determines the world's attitude toward us.

THE
ONE-HANDER'S
BOOK

EVERYDAY

In going about everyday living, it is helpful to keep objectives in mind and prepare ahead for each activity, so as to conserve time and energy. For example, you will want to keep currency, tickets, and keys at your fingertips as much as possible in your comings and goings. This will save your having to put packages down, for example, and rummaging through handbag or billfold to complete each transaction. Judge as closely as possible how much money you will need for a specific errand and carry that amount in a handy pocket. Keep your keys in a pocket or carry them in your hand while returning home so you will not have to set down your bundles and then lift them to get inside the door. These suggestions may sound trivial at first but you will come to see how much time and energy they will save.

Many times you will confront a closed door you want to enter while carrying something in your hand. Assuming you do not have

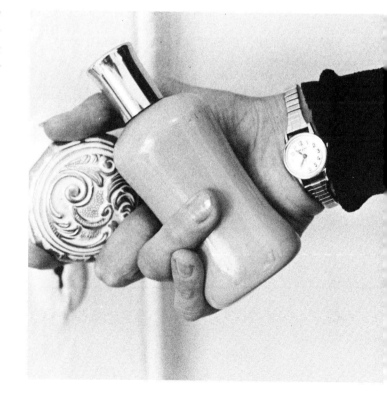

a pocket to slip the object into, you can turn the door knob this way: if the object is small enough, like a small bottle or a key case, you can hold it securely in the palm under your last two fingers while you turn the knob with your thumb and first two fingers. This may take some practice in the beginning. Or you may simply hold the object gently between your teeth to free your hand.

When carrying a larger bundle you can either place it on the floor or balance it on one knee before turning the knob. This is assuming that the door opens inward. Instead of entering face and bundle forward, you may find it easier to back into the door. If the door opens outward, place the bundle on the floor; your arm should be clear.

If you are a recent one-hander, the act of negotiating a newspaper, whether it be tabloid or standard size, on public transportation can be formidable. If the conveyance is bus, subway, train, or car, and one is seated, of course the lap will accommodate even the largest papers with no problem. But how does one stand, hold on, and negotiate a

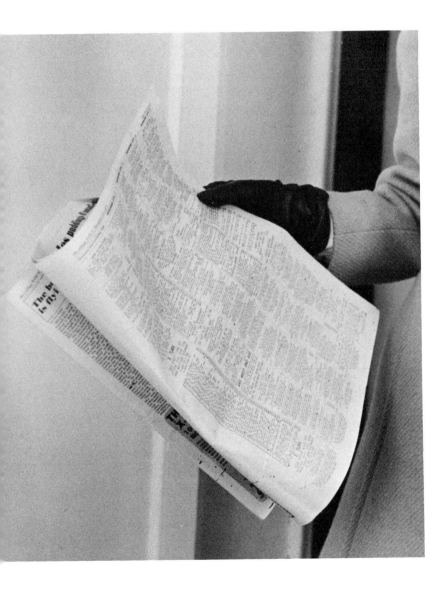

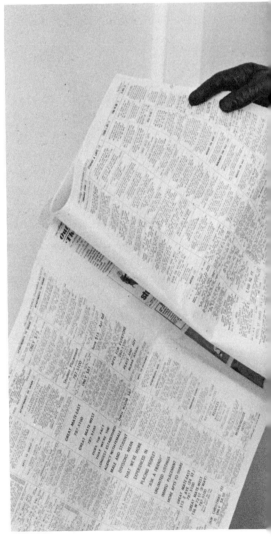

paper simultaneously? On subways this is accomplished during uncrowded hours by leaning against the doors or by circling your arm around the floor pole, which leaves your hand free. On some buses and most trains during rush hours it is possible to rivet your hip or thigh against a seat handle on the aisle for support, thus freeing your hand to turn the pages.

A small newspaper can be managed easily enough this way: release the pages with your thumb and let gravity "turn" them by slightly tilting the paper downward, to right or left, depending on which arm you use. Then, while you are bringing the paper upright, brush it slightly against your midsection, where your fingers pin it to complete the turn. The front and back pages of large newspapers can be read while standing on moving vehicles. If, however, you care to tackle the middle sheets of large-size papers in this situation, first gather the paper in a vertical fold, hold it securely, and thumb each page as described above.

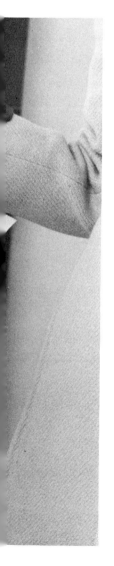
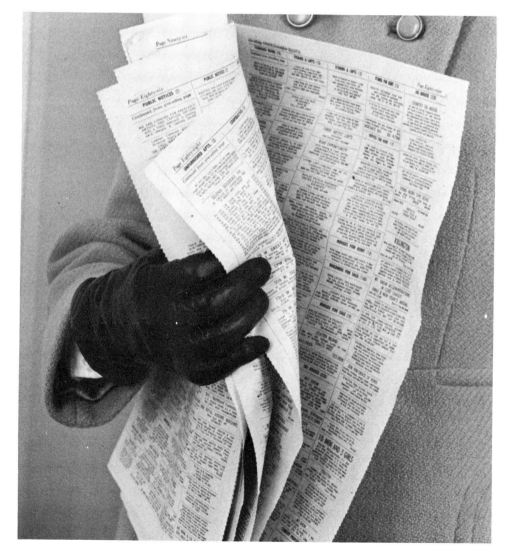

Most one-handers who smoke will probably use a cigarette lighter, but everyone should know how to light a match. Recent one-handers will find it simple, while seated, to place the closed matchbook under the side of their shoe to secure it for striking. Those who have more finger dexterity can secure the closed matchbook on any surface firmly under the last three fingers, holding the match between thumb and index finger and striking briskly. You will automatically pull your index finger in as the flame is lighted.

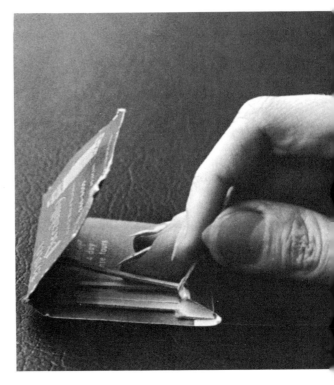

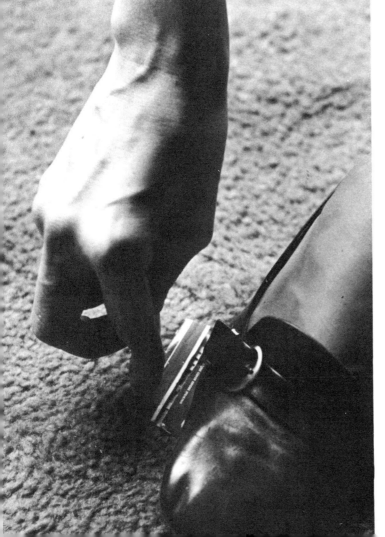

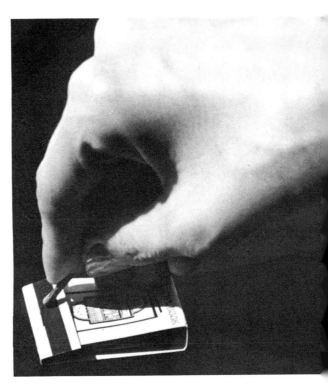

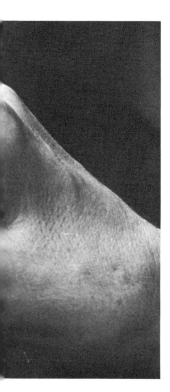

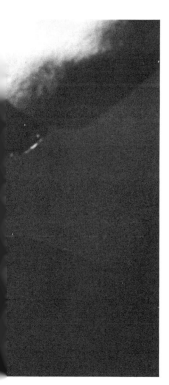

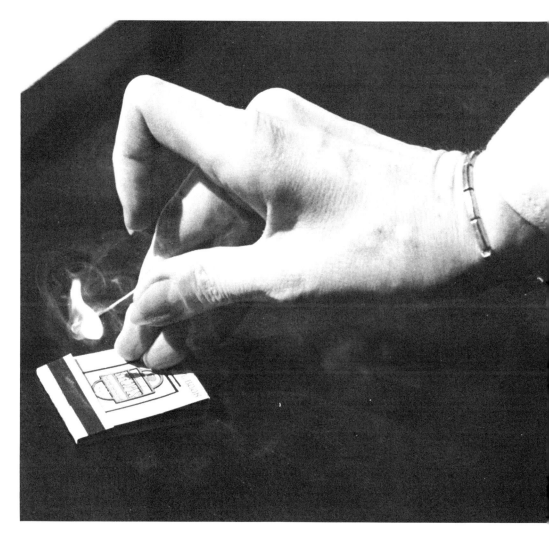

When having to make out checks, sign charge account sales slips, or write on other small surfaces in public, one-handers may be troubled by the sliding of these materials. If you have your other, or an artificial, arm, bring it up by means of your good hand onto the writing surface to create your own natural paperweight. If you have only one arm, you can fold half of the check or sales slip over the edge of the counter and hold it there with your midsection while you sign. Or you may allow the sales person, who is usually standing in attendance, to hold the slip steady. Sales people are often quick to anticipate this need. At home, of course, it is easy from either a standing or sitting position to use the other arm, if one has it, in the above fashion or a standard paperweight to hold down small writing surfaces.

We close this chapter with a suggestion of how to make use of some parts of the body to perform the "holding" activity that a second hand ordinarily would. These "holding" parts of the body are good to know about, for they come in handy at times and give us an out when we get into a jam. The areas that adapt themselves to the function of holding an object when the good hand is otherwise engaged are found: between the teeth; under the chin; under the armpit; between the knees; between the calves; and between the feet. If you need to free your hand quickly for a more immediate task while holding a package or two, secure that item, or items, at any of these areas that is appropriate and you are all set.

2

DRESSING AND GROOMING

A general rule of dressing for one-handers of both sexes is to "dress" the unusable arm and shoulder first before dressing the good arm. Either arm can be undressed first if the garment is a light one, such as a shirt or blouse. But the good arm must be undressed first if the garment is heavy, such as a coat, jacket, or rainwear.

Female one-handers need not assume they will have difficulty fastening underclothing. There are a number of shortcuts that will help. Bras and garter belts, for example, are first hooked in front, then turned around: hold one end of the garment to your waist at the side corresponding to your nonfunctioning arm; stand with this part of the body pressed against a dresser or chair to hold the end secure there. Now bring your good hand be-

hind you to pick up the other end of the bra or belt and fasten it in front. Some undergarments are designed to fasten in front, although they are not found everywhere.

Today's lightweight stretch, step-in girdles are not difficult to pull on with one hand, but it is sometimes advisable to buy a size larger than you normally wear. This not only makes the pulling on easier, but ensures a longer life for the garment because of less strain to the seams.

Most teenagers and slim women can shun girdles in favor of panty hose, which are a boon to one-handers because they eliminate the tugging on and the gartering. If it is a question of having to lose only a few pounds to be able to wear the panty hose, you would be well advised to do so.

If stockings have to be attached to garters, the hardest part is hooking the back ones, specifically the back garter for the leg that is opposite to the good arm. Front garters are hooked easily enough with one hand, as is the back garter on the leg corresponding to the good arm. To overcome the problem of attaching the back garter to the leg opposite the good arm without having to go into body contortions try this: garter the *back* of both stockings to the belt or girdle *before* putting the garment on; this can be done without difficulty because the front garters are unfastened. Unless the thighs are very large the stocking top will stretch enough to admit the leg. Otherwise try this: turn the trunk of the body toward the back of the leg that is opposite to the good arm—cross the good arm in front of the body to reach behind this leg—and extend it backward far enough to allow your hand to grip the garter firmly enough to fasten it. Whew! As you can see, attaching the garters beforehand is a simpler solution, and wearing panty hose that much easier!

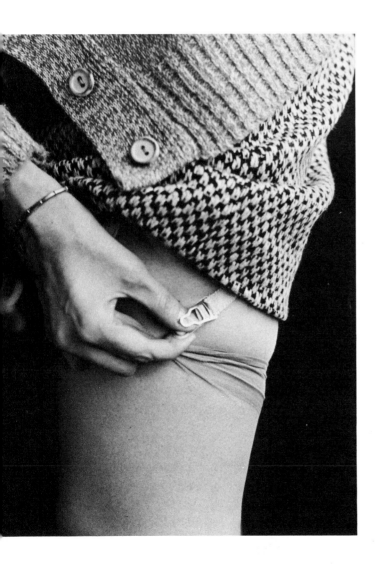
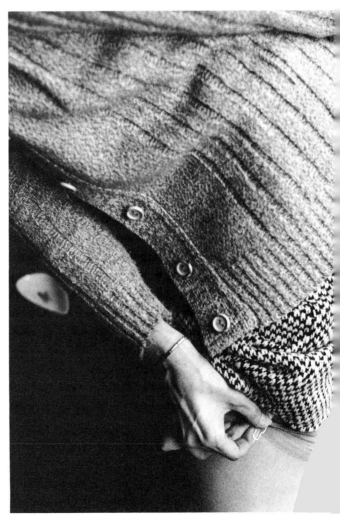

Getting into buttoned long-sleeved shirts and blouses without the aid of a second hand is fairly easy. Button or cuff-link the sleeve *before* putting your hand through, first cupping the hand to its smallest diameter. Women should not have trouble with this, but men with their larger hands may not maneuver as easily into their shirt sleeves. In this case the cuff button can be re-sewn closer to the cuff edge to enlarge the wrist opening (see chapter 9, Needle and Thread). To remove buttoned or nonbuttoned long-sleeved garments, first ease the garment off both shoulders, then reach behind your back with your good hand to pull the sleeve loose from the second hand (your good arm is still in its sleeve). Catch the loosened section of the garment between your knees to hold it secure while you pull your good arm out from the sleeve. This sleeve, of course, comes off inside out.

Cuff links in shirts or blouses sometimes have to be removed first before you can get your arm out (see above to get the arm through). Enlist your teeth to straighten the

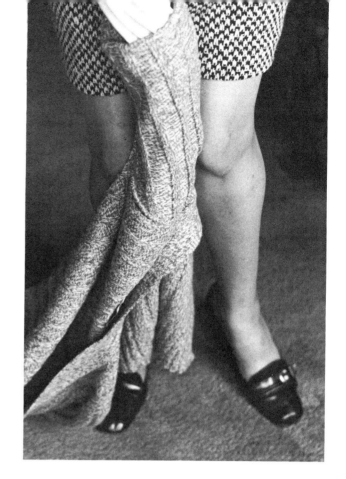

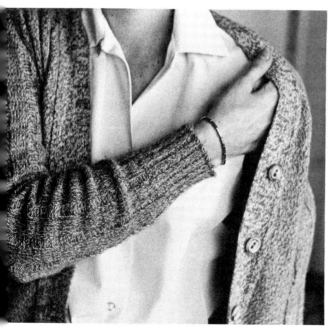

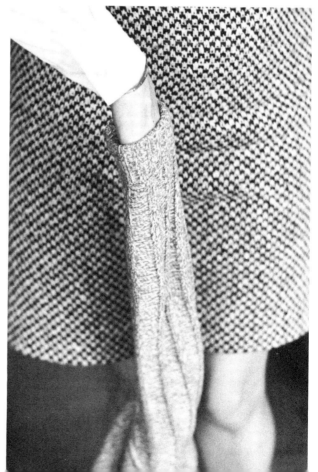

pin of the cuff link, then guide the pin through the cuff opening with your tongue. This is difficult in the beginning, to be sure, but it will come with practice and patience. (Girls will always remove their lipstick first!) Proceed in the manner just described to remove the arms from the sleeves.

Men and women whose second arm is shorter than the good arm can turn up the cuff on that long sleeve after it is buttoned so it does not hang to the fingers of the un-usable hand. The cuffs of long-sleeved dresses can be tucked under to the wrist length of the second hand and sewn in place. Again, where the sleeve opening is very wide re-sew the button closer to the cuff center, or take a tuck in the cuff to narrow it. Men's and women's suit jacket sleeves on the non-functioning arm can also be tucked under for shortening.

Women will do well to select clothing they can step into rather than over-the-head garments, which are harder to manage with one hand, and muss hair-do's besides. A tip for closing the back zipper is to double a piece of heavy thread through the opening in the zipper tab before getting into the dress. Step into the dress and pull the thread up your back to close the zipper. Another way to handle back zippers: be seated; bring the zipper halfway up from the waist, then stretch over your shoulder to complete the closing. There are zipper-closing aids on the market, too.

There is a technique for tying your shoes in which your foot substitutes for the second hand. (Recent one-handers may at first prefer to wear slip-on or buckle shoes.) Tying shoes can be mastered easily enough in this way: tighten the laces by pulling on both ends with your hand. Now cross the laces in an *X* shape

10

and pass one lace under, then through, the other to make the first knot. Tighten this half-knot by stepping on one of the laces with your second foot and pulling the other lace in the opposite direction with your hand. Now loop one side of the lace around your index finger and center this half-loop in the middle of the knot, holding it there with your middle finger. Release the second lace from under your foot, and with your index and thumb work this lace around and under the first loop (still held by the middle finger) to form the final loop of the tie. Tighten the laces by inserting your middle finger through one loop and pulling the second loop in the opposite direction with your index finger and thumb. Your shoelace is securely tied.

If you have to tie shoes on toddlers, you can use your teeth to pull and hold the other lace in the same way that your other foot maneuvers this, as described (see also chapter 10, Baby and Child Care).

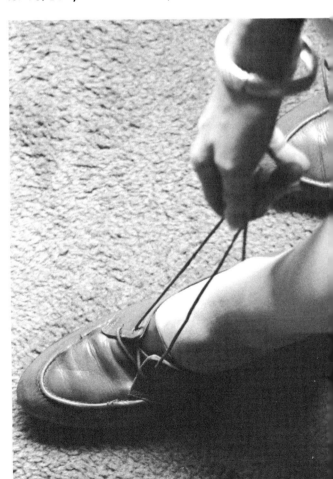

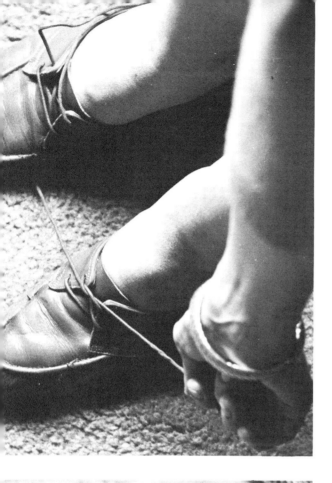
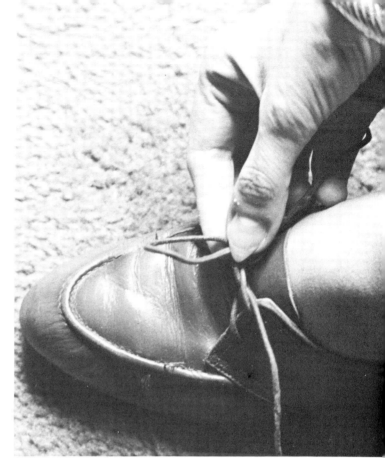
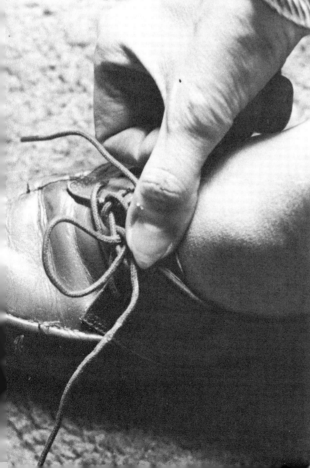
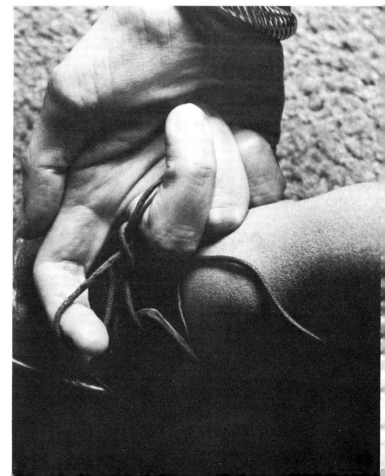

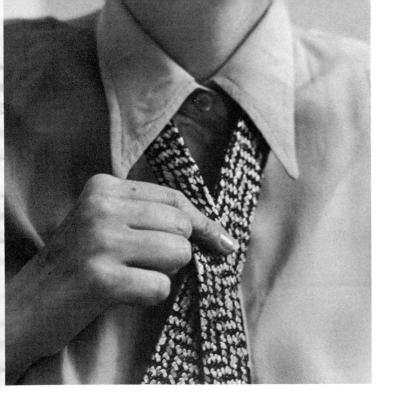

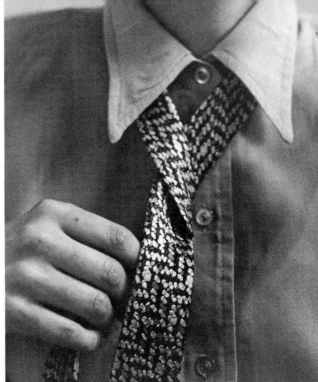

Men can knot their ties with one hand in this manner: secure the tie under your shirt collar, allowing one end to hang longer, and hold both ends of the tie at the center of your lower throat. Cross one end over the other— once, then twice. Now take up the top end and tuck it under, then bring it through the large loop of tie around your neck. Insert this same tie end down through the small loop, just formed, which now becomes the tie knot. Pull down firmly on this same end to tighten the knot. The knot is now positioned at your upper chest; raise it in position by grasping both ends of the tie under your last two fingers and inching the knot upwards to the throat with your thumb and middle fingers. Your tie is as secure as if it were tied with two hands.

Men can also buy pre-knotted ties and bow ties that clip on the collar and eliminate

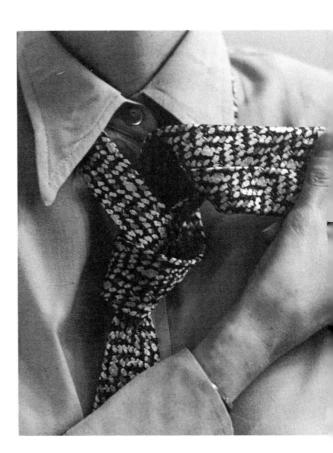

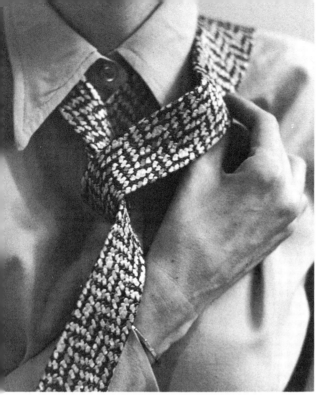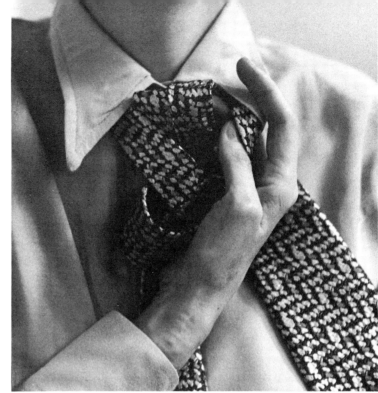
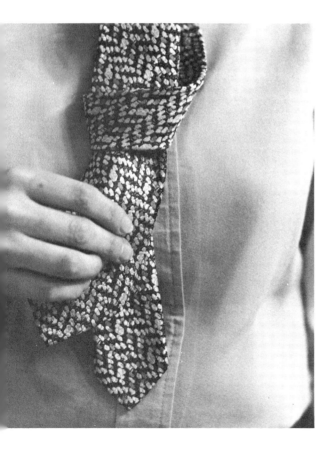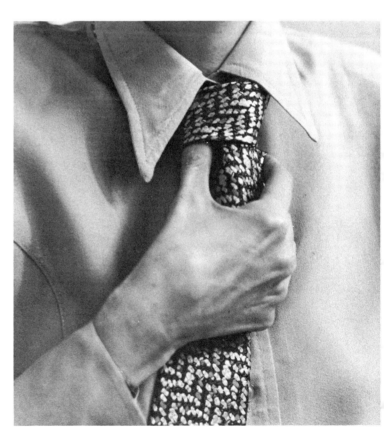

the need for hand-tying. There is not the variety of pattern and color with the clip-ons, however, and they are not found everywhere.

Male one-handers who wear suspenders can work these easily by first attaching the back suspenders before getting into the trousers. It is simple then to hook the front straps.

One-handers should have no trouble putting on gloves. First glove your unusable hand, if you have one, in the usual way. (For the sake of appearance you are encouraged to glove even an artificial hand—see also chapter 5, Caring for the Good Hand.) Pick up the other glove by inserting your fingers into its cuff, then bring it to your midsection to hold it steady while you "wiggle" your hand in. You can work your fingers down completely into the glove by pushing on the crotch of each finger along the edge of any suitable object at hand, for example, the back of a chair.

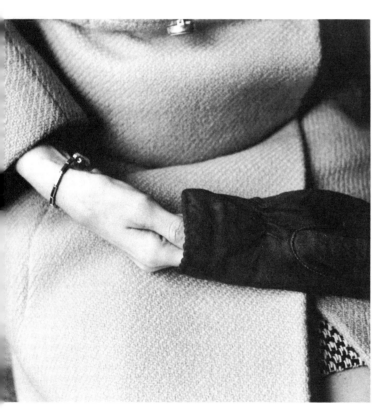 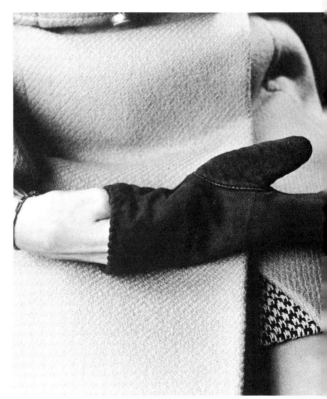

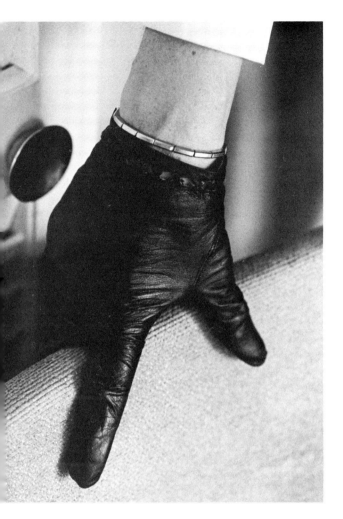
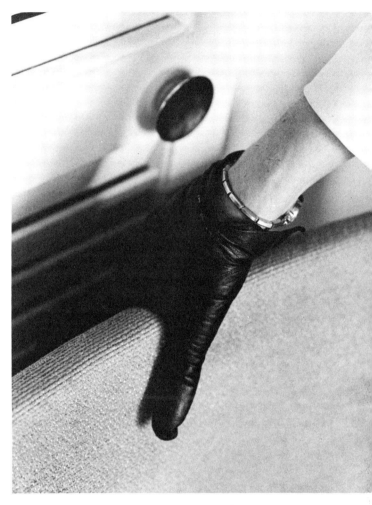

Women can fasten costume jewelry unassisted. Stand before a mirror and hook chokers and necklaces in front before turning them around. (You can steady the eye section of the fastener by resting it against your lower neck before attaching the hook.) If the good hand is small enough, you may be able to hook bracelets and wriggle your hand in.

Otherwise purchase the bangle-type bracelet or ones with a tension band that snaps closed. Perform this by slipping into the bracelet, supporting your wrist against your midsection, then stand close up to a wall or any stationary object and apply pressure to the clasp to lock the bracelet.

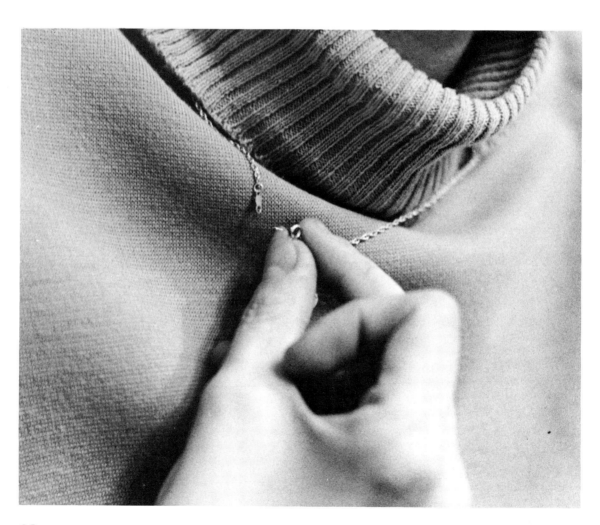

Clip-on earrings are by far the most practical for one-handers, although you can handle the screw type this way: working on the ear that corresponds to the good hand, insert the lobe between the earring metal. Press the earring to the outer lobe with your middle finger; now that the earring is secured the thumb and index finger tighten the screw. Fastening the far earring proceeds the same way, with the exception that the index finger presses the earring to the lobe while the thumb and middle finger tighten the screw. Fastening earrings to pierced ears is done by pressing the earlobe firmly to the head with the middle finger. This widens the opening enough to slip the wire in with your thumb and index finger.

Women whose nonfunctioning arm has the same appearance as the good one and has sensation as well may like to wear rings and/or bracelets on this hand and arm. This is all right providing the jewelry is worn loosely enough so as not to impair the circulation of this arm. If the nonfunctioning arm is shorter and thinner, however, wearing costume jewelry accents the arm contours, which many women might wish to avoid.

Expansion watch bands are easier for one-handers to put on and remove than strap bands, which we do not describe here because they are not likely to be preferred. Place the watch on a dresser or table top and cup your fingers inside the band to expand it over your knuckles. Now either hold your hand to your midsection and "roll" the watch, face up, over your hand into place at your wrist, or catch the band under a small round knob of the type found on bureau drawers

and pull the band gently into place. The knob here does the work of a second hand. Remove the watch by performing the reverse of either of these two methods. To set and wind your watch, first hold it to your midsection to steady it. Incidentally, you might buy an expansion band a little small so the constant stretching occasioned by getting into and out of it does not loosen the band so much that it slides around on the wrist.

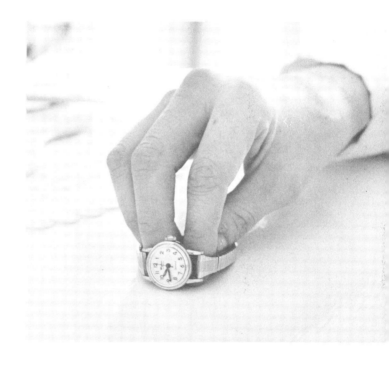

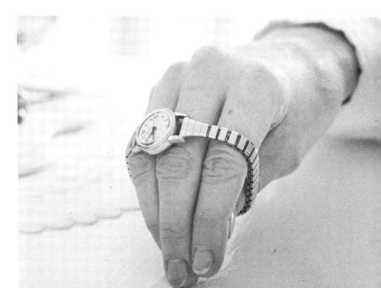

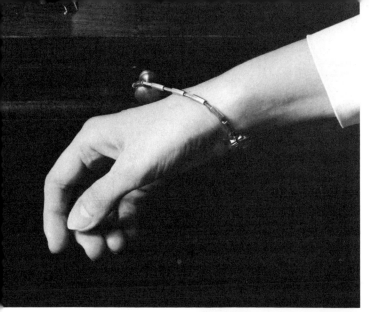

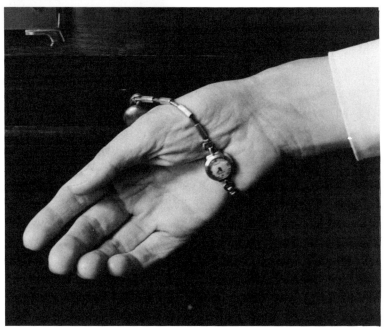

18

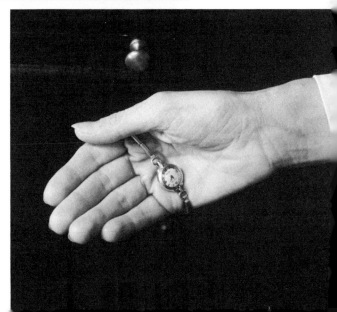

Men and women who wear beret-style or close-fitting hats can put them on this way: place the beret on your head at the tip of your forehead, leaving a small section of brim slightly lower over the forehead. Now stand close up to a wall or open door and press your forehead to it to catch the brim and secure it. The wall becomes your second "hand," allowing your good hand to position the beret in place at the angle you wear it.

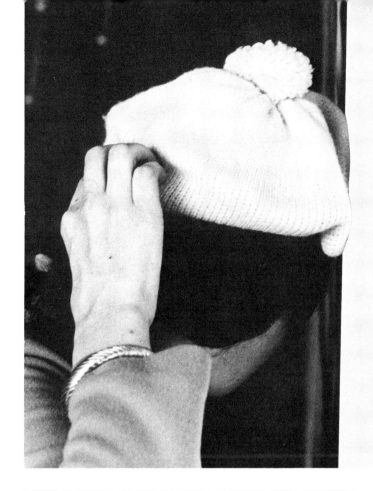

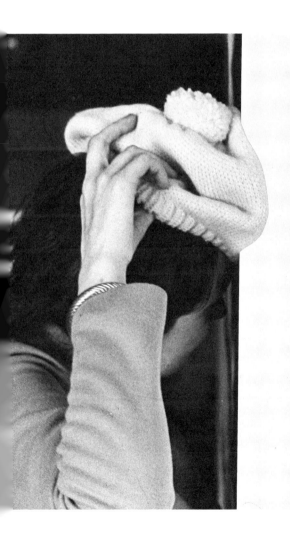

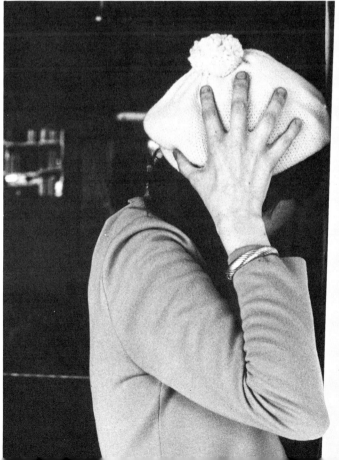

Kerchief tying is easy with one hand. Bring the kerchief over your head, centering it so both ends hang evenly. Hold one end between your index and middle finger and catch the other end with your fourth finger. Now cross the first end over, then up through the second to make the first knot. Tighten the knot by holding one end between your teeth while you pull on the other. Repeat this step for the second knot and your kerchief is secure.

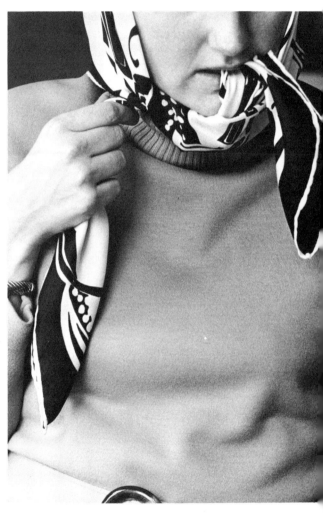

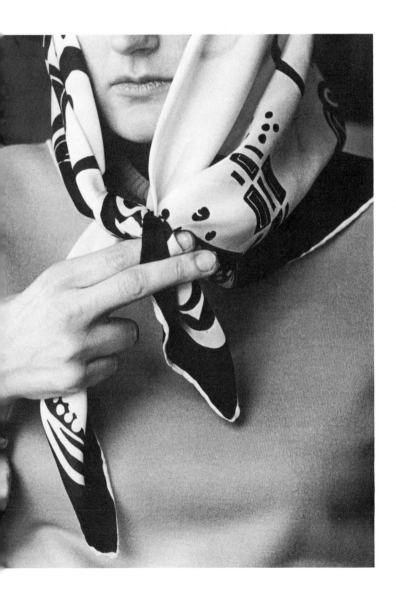

Swimmers may have difficulty putting on a bathing cap with one hand because tight rubber is not easy to handle. Purchase a cap that is one size larger than your head size. You can put it on from a sitting or standing position this way: if you are sitting in the sand or on a dock, for example, hold the cap firmly by the back edge, in the center, and place the front edge at about eyebrow level. Now gently slide the cap backwards over your forehead until the front edge reaches just below your hairline. Raise your knee and bring your head down to it to hold the front of the cap secure there. Now you can pull the cap back over your head. When the cap is on, push the remaining hairs under. From a standing position you can use almost anything that is stationary (a wall or door, for example) to brace your head against while you pull the cap on, in the manner described above for beret hats. If this technique defeats you the first several tries, be assured that it will come with practice.

One side of the outer clothing of one-handers wears out more quickly than the other side. By virtue of holding and carrying packages on one side, inserting the hand in and out of one pocket, and general friction to the clothing on the side of the good arm, which is natural to one-handers, one side shows soil and wear while the side of the nonfunctioning arm shows little or no wear. This can be a problem that sends us to the cleaners more often—contributing further to the wear! Keep your clothing from wearing prematurely by spraying garments when they are new or fresh from the cleaners with a fabric protector on those areas that take the heaviest wear: the cuff and sleeve (front and back) of the good arm, and the front and side of the garment corresponding to the good arm. Particularly, spray light-colored summer and winter clothing.

Women can get into the habit of carrying a mini shopping bag for those little parcels that one picks up almost daily, instead of carrying them in a bag in their arm against the clothing. Newspapers should be carried in a clear plastic wrapper. Of course greater shopping will require larger shopping bags. To some extent, packages and bundles will naturally come in contact with clothing, but we can reduce considerably the wear caused by this.

Around the house women may want to wear a smock to keep their street and/or house dresses from wearing or soiling on one side.

Men will find the friction centers on their suits and sport clothes are the pockets, inside and out, the jacket cuff, the button area, and the elbow of the good arm. This can be remedied by reinforcing these areas with extra cloth or sewing an elbow patch on sport jackets (sew one on the other sleeve to keep it uniform). A tailor, a wife, or a mother may be needed here.

You will be able to keep yourself well groomed with one hand without requiring help from anyone.

Your shower and bath proceed in the usual manner up to the point where you wash your good arm. To do this, first place your foot corresponding to the arm up on the edge of the tub. Place the soaped washcloth on the lower thigh (which is now bent). Move your arm up, down, and around over the cloth for a scrubbing. You can dry your arm the same way. To wash under your good arm, wad the washcloth into a ball and apply it to the armpit with circular motions. You are best advised to use a long-handled brush to wash your back, although you can also accomplish this by squeezing the soapy cloth over each shoulder, then bringing your arm behind and up the middle of your back and soaping that section. To dry your back, fold a medium-sized bath towel in half and grip the corners firmly in your hand; now sling the middle portion over first one shoulder, then the other.

There should be a rubber mat on the bottom of your tub. You will appreciate one particularly after a bath, when you rise from a kneeling position. This safety tip will prevent your slipping. You may find a shower caddy is most useful for holding all your bathing essentials (shampoo, soap, bath oils, washcloth, brush, etc.) within hand's reach in one place, so you will not have to stoop at every turn.

Women and girls who wish to use a depilatory for the underarm area can apply this to the pit of the good arm by the same method described previously for bathing this area. If the nonfunctioning arm is not rigid it can be propped on top of a bureau or up against the bathroom wall before applying the depilatory; if the arm is rigid use your fingers to apply lotion to the side of the armpit.

Both men and women would do well to take advantage of the many grooming aids that come in spray containers. This is by far the quickest and neatest method one-handers have to apply deodorants, body powder, dry shampoo, hair coloring, colognes, depilatories, shaving creams, etc., without spills or waste. Further grooming conveniences are offered by spray shoe polish, spot remover, and fabric protector (on shirts, dresses, blouses, etc.). Form the habit early: spray—and you won't spill!

Feminine one-handers can perfume the wrist of their good hand this way: before dressing spray a mist of cologne or perfume to the skin of your midsection on the side that corresponds to your hand; quickly rub your wrist and forearm into the mist for a thorough application.

Men will discover that shaving with one hand takes no more finesse than shaving with two. This is equally true for the standard or the electric razor shave. The facial area is tightened by puffing the cheeks with air and holding them that way as you apply the razor. Tighten the chin area by sharply pulling in your lower lip. To shave between the folds of skin at the neck, crane your head up and backward to tighten this area enough to prevent razor nicks.

To wash your comb and brush, either soak them first in warm sudsy water, or run the comb through the brush, secured in the basin or at sink edge as described for nail cleaning (see chapter 5, Caring for the Good Hand).

3

HAIR STYLING AND CARE

Washing, brushing, and combing hair need not be a problem for one-handers. Women with particularly thick hair might do well to use a shampoo brush to make washing easier. Hair can be towel-dried, turban style, or blown dry with a hair dryer. Women may prefer these methods to hand-drying the hair with a heavy towel. Girls with long hair, whether thick or fine, will find it practical to use a cream rinse or other hair conditioner before combing through wet hair. Damp, tangled hair is a trial even for two-handers, so this prevention is worth the attention.

One-handers can arrange different hair styles by themselves especially if hair length is medium to long and the texture is fairly straight. Naturally, short hair is easiest to maintain. Before you begin to set or style your hair, place a mirror in front and one in back to guide you. Pin out of the way hair you are not working with.

If hair is long, you have a choice of using hair rollers, to turn the ends up or under, or bobby pins for curly styles. (Both these techniques are for setting the ends of the hair— not the hair at the crown.) Hair rollers will be easier to use until you have built up enough finger dexterity for the bobby-pin setting. The rollers simplest to use are the self-adhering ones that grip the hair with tiny nylon projections and hold them securely to the head without your having to add clips. This type of hair roller is used in the techniques here.

Some of these techniques for setting and styling the hair will seem complex in the reading, especially for the recent one-hander, but with practice they will become automatic.

To turn the ends under with rollers, first slip your index finger through the roller and, starting at the upper strands of the sectioned hair, gather this hair between your middle and fourth fingers. Now bring the roller finger in toward your cheek and brush the roller through this sectioned hair in a downward motion almost to the hair ends. With your middle finger scoop the lower ends up under the roller. The hair will stick to it and allow your thumb and index fingers to roll the curler under. To set the back of your hair, place the roller under the sectioned hair strand and press your hair to it. Work the hair under the roller with your thumb and roll it under into place.

To turn the ends up, take a section of hair and place the roller over the strand of hair just above the ends. Press the roller into the hair, supporting it against your neck, or with shorter hair, against the lower jaw. Your hair will stick to the roller, allowing your fingers to work the ends up over the roller. Simply roll the curler into place.

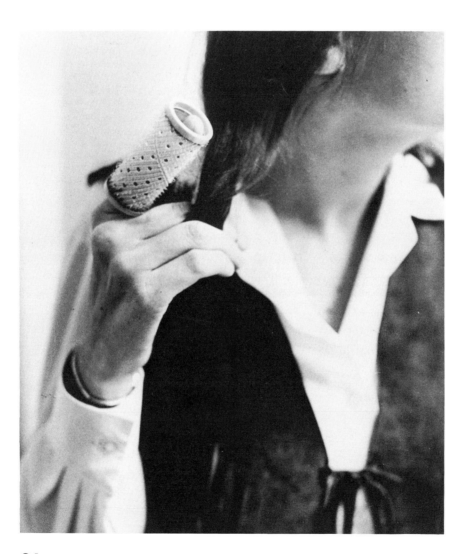

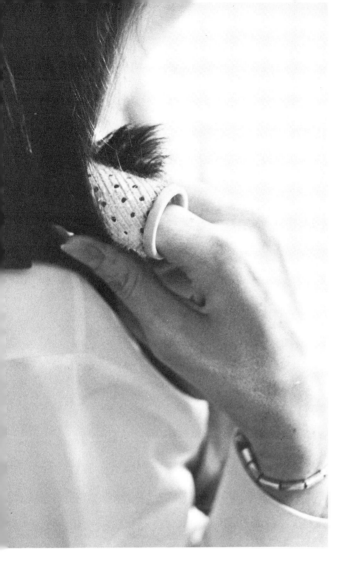

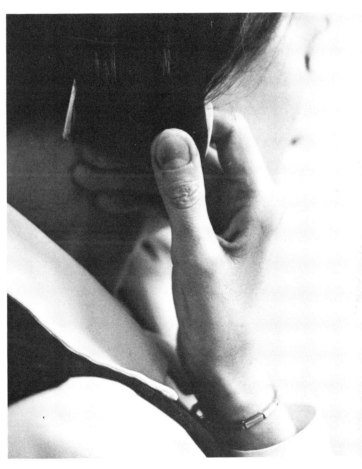

Learning to set your hair with bobby pins will require some patience in the beginning. The trick is to manipulate the bobby pin on your finger at the same time you are forming the curl. It is done this way: prop the pin up on your dresser top or against your midsection, closed end down. Slide your thumb into the pin to open it. This position of the pin on your thumb tip is maintained to the completion of the curl. With thumb tip and middle finger grasp a section of hair at the crown and slide your middle and fourth fingers down the strand to about one-half inch from the ends. Now position your index finger at about ear level at a right angle to your head. Your middle finger guides the hair halfway around the index finger in a circular position. Your thumb tip presses this hair strand to your head as the fourth finger slips into the curl's center. Around this finger and thumb, your index and little fingers press the curl to your head and release the fourth finger. The hardest part is over! Your middle and fourth fingers now hold the completed curl in place while your thumb slips the opened bobby pin through the curl.

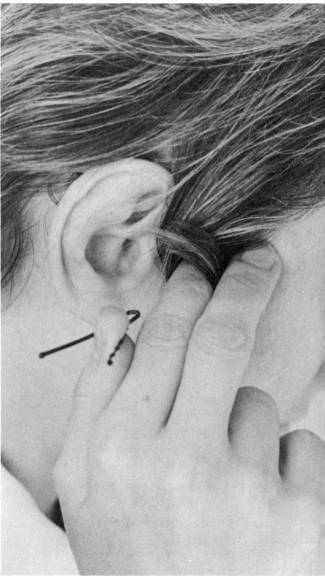

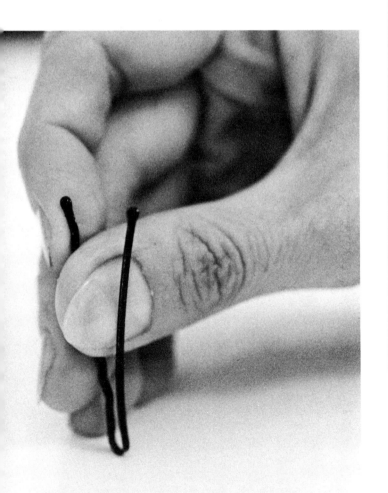

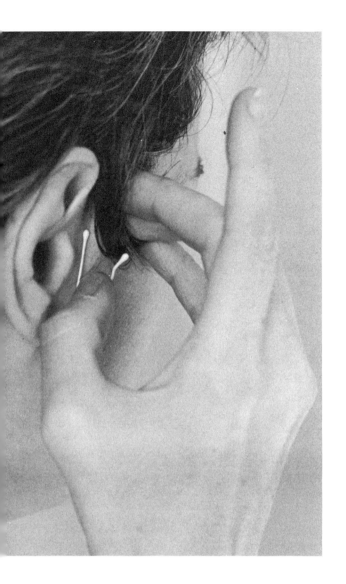

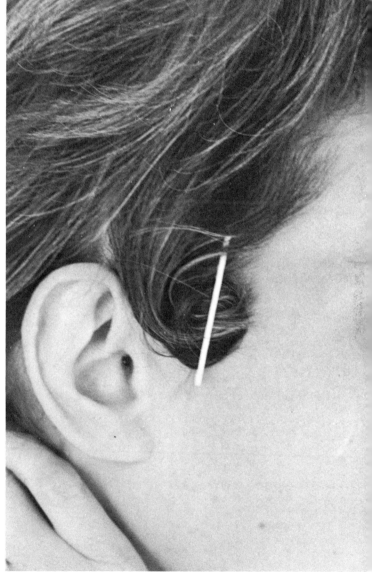

27

You can even tease your own hair with one hand providing it is medium to long in length. In a seated position bend your head down to your knees. Catch and hold a section of hair at a time between your knees and proceed to tease-comb that section, working from hair ends to scalp. You can tease the sides as easily as the crown simply by turning your head to either side and securing that section of hair between your knees.

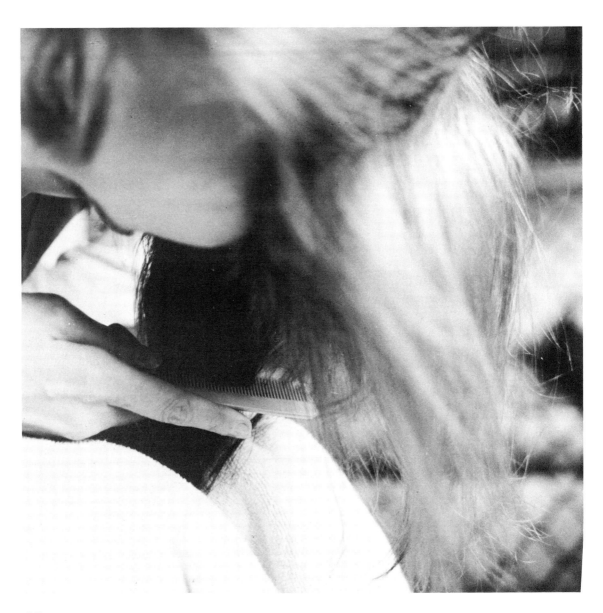

Now for hair styles:

To achieve a ponytail (high at the crown), lie down face up on a flat surface or bed and comb your hair away from the nape of the neck and forehead in a straight line to the hair ends; the hair should look like an open fan. Now tighten a rubber band around your thumb and first three fingers. Slip the thumb under and the fingers on top of the hair at your crown, tilting your head backwards to assist the motion. With your index and middle fingers, work your hair through the band and voila! you have a secure ponytail.

(See next page on how to tighten rubber band)

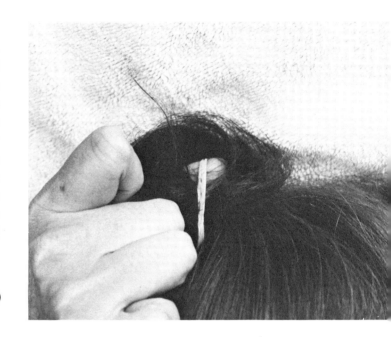

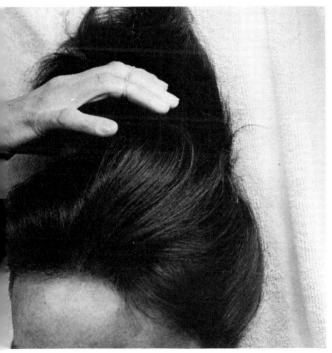

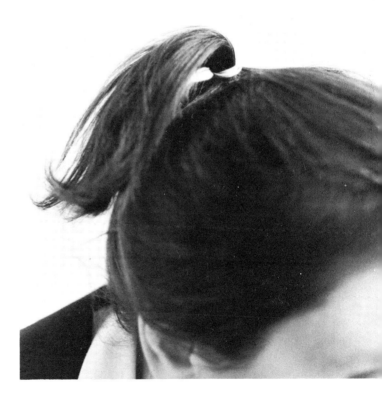

The low, neck ponytail takes the same technique with the rubber band and only requires that you gather the hair between thumb and middle fingers at the back of your neck and pull the hair through the band with your index finger.

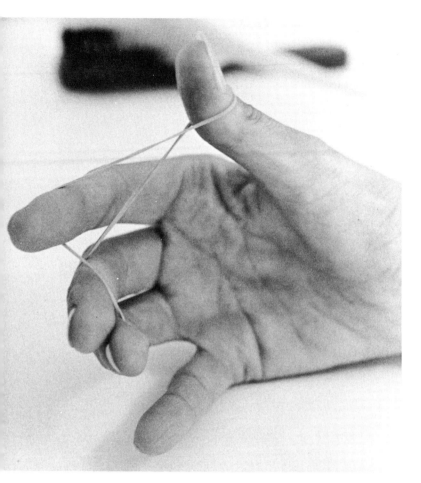

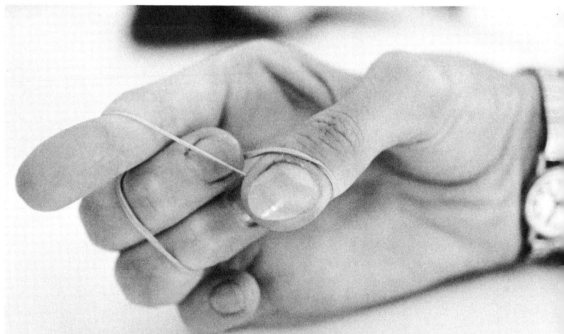

To make a twist, place your thumb between an opened bobby pin and gather your hair at the back of your neck. With your thumb and middle finger, hold the hair and grip it between your palm and the middle and fourth fingers. Now lower your thumb and forethumb down over this thatch of hair, turning it under and around your index finger. The middle finger anchors it here. Turn your hand slightly toward your head, pressing the newly twisted hair to your head with the aid of the forethumb. Now release all your fingers except the thumb and knead the hair toward your head into a sausage shape. This places your middle and fourth fingers back inside the twist in about the center of the back of your head. Straighten your thumb; press the twist toward your head and anchor it with the forethumb. Bring your fingers out (the twist is made) and press this rolled hair to your head with your middle and fourth fingers. Now pivot your hand around so the opened bobby pin on your thumb is facing the rear crown of your head. Ease the bobby pin into the top part of the twist, shifting the index and middle fingers to admit it; push the pin with your thumb as far down into the twist as it will go. Bring your hand away and proceed to pin the bottom end of the twist in place. Anchor it with as many pins as it needs and finish with a hair spray. This process is difficult at first but it will come with some practice. The many compliments I receive on my one-hand twists, done this way, prove that it does work.

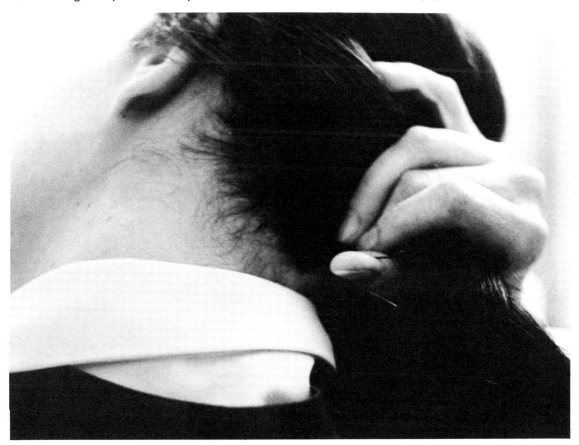

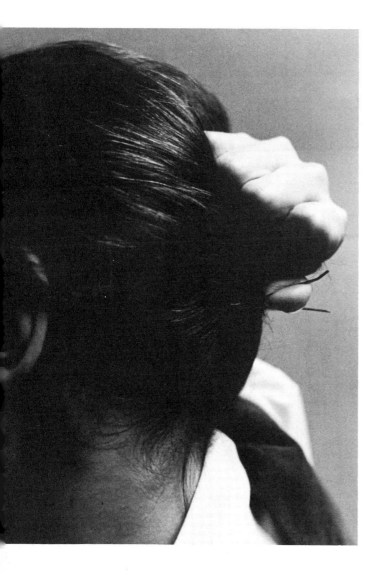

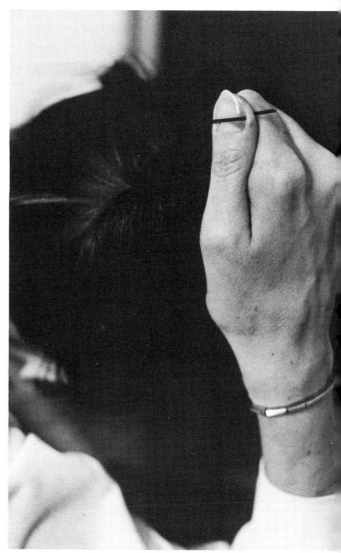

32

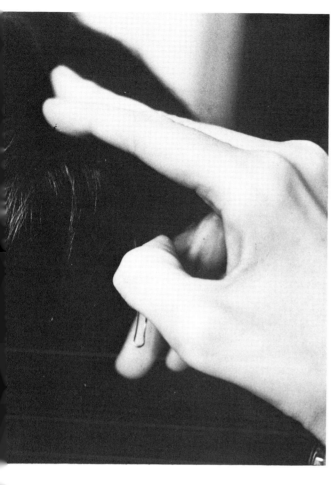

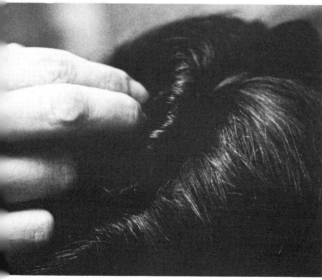

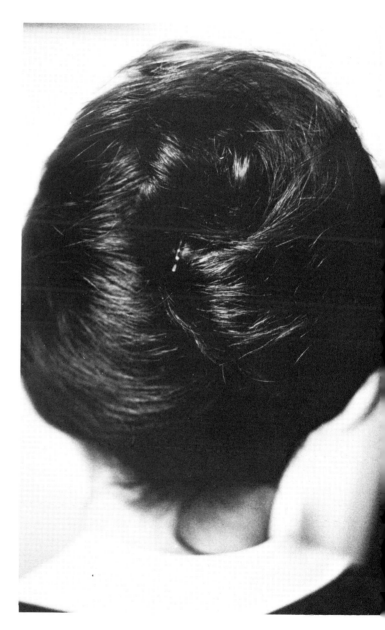

If you want to create the bouffant look of a high crown with back hair combed straight, try this: comb your hair away from the face and behind your ears. Place an opened bobby pin over your thumb and extend your middle finger at a right angle to the temple slightly behind your ear. Now run this finger through to the scalp, up the side of your head to the crown. You will have gathered up the top hair on one side. Transfer your thumb to this spot to keep the hair intact. Now the rest of your hand is free to pivot across the top of your head to the other temple, where your middle finger gathers up the top hair from the other side and brings it back to meet the thumb. You are now holding between your forethumb and middle fingers at the crown of your head a thatch of top hair. Work your four fingers under this hair securing it against your palm; your thumb is extended. Work the hair under your index finger with your forethumb and hold this piece to your head with the middle finger. Turn your hand in slightly toward your head to accommodate your thumb with its opened bobby pin. Simply slip the pin through this knot of hair and insert a few more pins to secure it. For best results the knot should be centered rather high at the back of the crown. The hair in back is combed straight down and you have another attractive hair style.

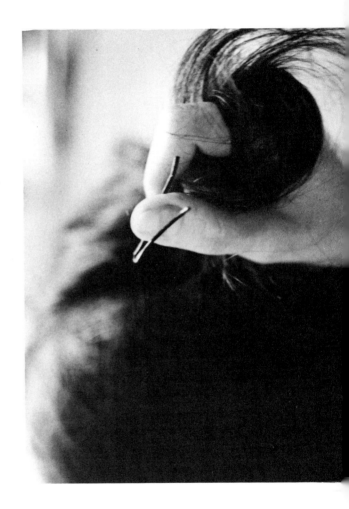

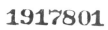

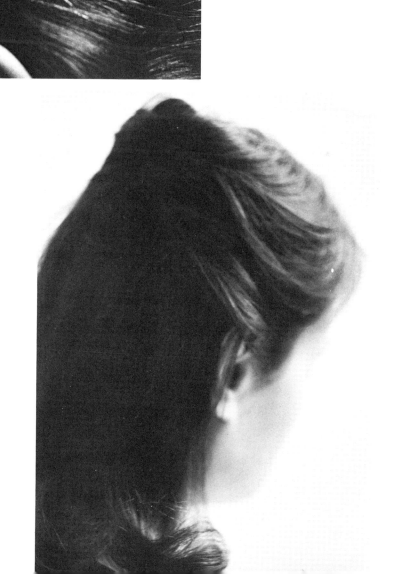

35

Wigs and hairpieces are worn for every imaginable social situation today. Recent one-handers may find them particularly convenient until they have adjusted to managing their hair with one hand. Wigs can be brushed and styled on a wig stand which has a suction base. Insert hatpins through the styrofoam wig stand at the crown, sides, and back to anchor it. This will steady it while you comb and style. Wigs can be put on the same way as the beret (see chapter 2, Dressing and Grooming.) Fastening hairpieces in place requires much pinning, easily managed with one hand. Again, use a mirror in back to guide you.

4

FASHION-WISE

The one-hander's wardrobe will not differ significantly from the two-hander's, with a few exceptions. Where there is deformity of arm or shoulder we learn to understate rather than emphasize our clothing in those areas. All of us have good and bad features, which we dress up or down. Very few people have perfect figures; and almost everyone has need to camouflage some physical flaw, however small, sometime during his or her life.

Women and girls with an arm and/or shoulder deformity will be more selective in buying their clothing. One-handers whose unusable arm has the same appearance as the good one need not vary their style of dressing. Some one-handers may not be sensitive to their appearance, and therefore feel no need to camouflage. Others may be guided by a few basic wardrobe tips; these are merely suggestions, however, for one-handers are encouraged to experiment with their own ideas about styles and design.

1. Avoid short sleeves because they set off the contour of the arm. *Do* wear sleeveless fashions, especially in lighter shades if you are fair, as they do not set off the shape of the arm, surprising as this may seem. Black, brown, navy, and other dark-colored sleeveless outfits are becoming to dark-skinned persons. But these colors draw attention to the arm contours of fair-skinned persons. Raglan and cap-sleeves are not flattering if there is arm deformity. Long and three-quarter sleeves are most comfortable, particularly in cool weather.

2. Avoid seamless shoulder apparel, as in raglan or dolman sleeve. Set-in sleeves disguise shoulder irregularity best. Buy coats, suits, jackets, sweaters, dresses, blouses, robes, and sporty tops that have set-in sleeves.

3. Insert shoulder pads in the set-in sleeves of your lightweight garments, including blouses, house robes, and summer jackets. Padding smooths over an irregular

shoulder and gives a more balanced look to these contours.

4. Become aware of pockets; they are extremely practical as well as comfortable for one-handers. In all your clothes shopping, from house robes to evening gowns, select items of clothing that have pockets, and make this a prerequisite to the purchase.

Pockets free your hand in an instant; they are a place in which to slip your unusable hand when dashing for a train or for warmth in cold weather. Naturally, coats and suits should have them. Note that bucket pockets are not flattering to one-handers who have an arm deformity. Side pockets or front ones slit on the diagonal are becoming.

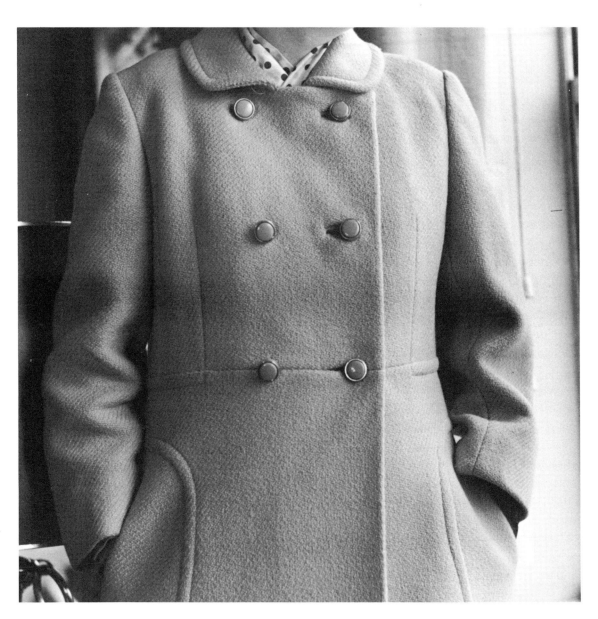

It is possible to camouflage the non-functioning, malformed arm even in a sleeveless outfit. Wear a very full skirt that has a side pocket and slip your hand into it. The blouse should match your skin coloring. Teenagers, who might feel self-conscious about their arm at first, will welcome this suggestion.

One-handers with a shoulder deformity or generally narrow shoulders will find that outfits with V-neck collars tend to make small shoulders appear larger. The boat-neck collar is a becoming style for small shoulders but should be worn in dark colors only because white and pastels in this style reveal shoulder contours. Turtlenecks tend to accentuate narrow and/or irregular shoulders. Of course, avoid halter tops if there is a problem shoulder.

If you are fair and have a malformed arm or shoulder, select your bathing suit in a lighter shade; also avoid those with dark or very thin shoulder straps. One-handers with dark skin who have an arm or shoulder irregularity should select a bathing suit that closely matches their skin coloring, and avoid white suits and thin shoulder straps. This applies also to sleeveless blouses, sundresses, and all outer clothing. By diminishing color contrast of clothing to skin tone, less attention is called to an irregularity. By selecting garments with wider shoulder straps we can partially conceal a malformed shoulder. Nightwear and undergarments of assorted styles and colors can, of course, be worn.

Evening clothes, such as prom gowns and more sophisticated formal attire, require careful selection. If there is an arm or shoulder deformity we would most likely want these areas covered. Strapless and sleeveless attire would be avoided by most one-handers. Happily, long-sleeved evening wear is always in fashion. Evening pants suits, gowns with long, flowing sleeves, and jumpsuits are a boon to one-handers. Most of these styles can be worn as they come from the rack, except perhaps for turning under the cuff of the unusable hand or inserting shoulder pads. Other styles, such as the Grecian gown, may require an extra layer of chiffon draping over the shoulders. The Indian sari worn over the choti or blouse with long sleeves is perfect for one-handers. Surprisingly, many evening fashions are designed with one or two side pockets.

If your are anticipating an important engagement such as a high school prom, a college weekend, or a formal ball, and you have sufficient time, you may prefer to have a gown made up for you to your own specifications and design. More and more people are sewing nowadays and you might find just the person in your neighborhood to do this for about the same price as, or less than, a store-bought gown.

Can one-handers wear evening gloves with their formal clothes? Yes—if there is no deformity or if you have a well-formed artificial arm or hand. Otherwise, you might simply carry gloves or not use them at all. Gloves, like short sleeves, call attention to arm contours. A suggestion is to carry them in summer, wear them in winter, and do either of these for evening wear according to the appearance of the arm.

Using a shawl or stole for evening or dressy occasions may feel slightly uncomfortable to one-handers. The reason for this is we must simultaneously hold both ends of the shawl in place and secure the second arm if we do not want it to hang loosely. If we add a clutch purse to the costume, things can become "un-handle-able." We can skirt this problem either by leaving the purse at home and simply carry a slim pouch in the pocket of the gown or by having an evening purse with a long chain handle and slipping this over the wrist of either the good or the nonfunctioning arm. Or, we can select a cape instead of a shawl. Most capes hook or button in the front to leave our hand free. To wear the shawl or stole successfully, one-handers must remember not to use the good

arm simultaneously for social activities such as hand-shaking and smoking, but to wait either until they are seated or have removed the stole and secured it over their good arm before engaging in these activities.

The poncho is another garment that offers a good camouflage to one-handers with an arm deformity. If there is shoulder deformity wear a bulky sweater or a blouse with shoulder pads beneath it to smooth the shoulder contour. In winter weather wear a heavy sweater under the poncho for warmth and to aid the circulation of the second, nonfunctioning arm.

Where there is a second or artificial arm

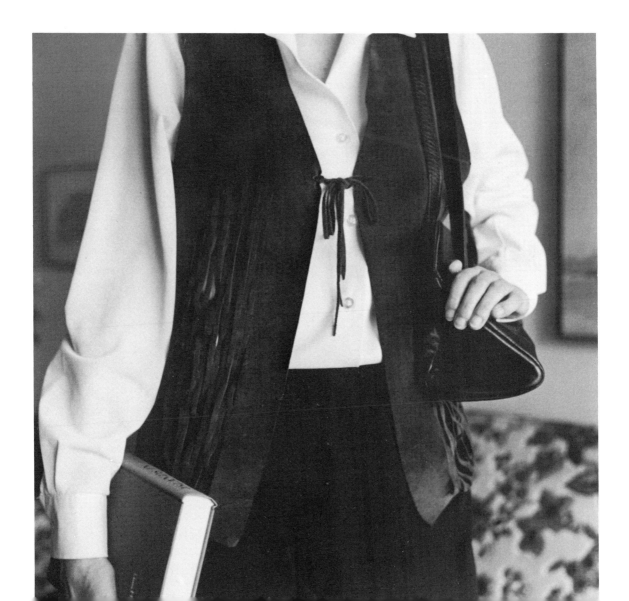

one-handers may find it very practical to carry a shoulder bag over the shoulder of the unusable arm. This leaves the good hand free, looks natural, and is quite comfortable on your daily rounds. Simply slip it over that shoulder and rest your hand on the top of the bag. This tends to work better with lightweight clothing than on winter coats, where the added weight of the coat sleeve pulls the shoulder strap off the shoulder. Using a shoulder bag this way is enthusiastically recommended for comfort and convenience.

Men have less of a clothing "problem," principally because most men are by nature less concerned with camouflage than women are. Many men would probably wear short sleeves in summer whether or not they have an arm deformity or an artificial arm. Other men will stay with long-sleeved shirts all summer, especially those who work in air-conditioned surroundings. If the shoulder is malformed and appearance is of more than ordinary concern, men may prefer more starch in their summer shirts or even having shoulder pads sewn in to create a more balanced shoulder contour. Starched cotton shirts camouflage a bad shoulder better than shirts made from synthetics. Some men may prefer extra padding in the shoulders of their summer suits as well.

5

CARING FOR THE GOOD HAND

Your good hand and arm present a great challenge in grooming because they are somewhat inaccessible and may show wear prematurely because they are exposed to everything and perform myriad tasks unassisted. To counteract this we acquire a new respect for the hand and arm which takes the form of proper grooming care, protection from strong cleaning solutions and cold weather, intervals of rest, and hand and arm massage. It also takes the form of vigilance in keeping the hand in good working order by preventing cuts, bruises, sprains, burns, swellings, and fractures.

The following suggestions for good care are designed to help keep the hand working smoothly to perform for a lifetime the tasks of daily living. If you have your second hand you will give it much of the attention that you give your good hand: washing it, applying lotion, manicuring, and protecting it from cold.

It is, of course, easier to care for the hand and nails of the nonfunctioning hand.

Washing the good hand is accomplished more easily if you have a second hand to assist. In this case, hold a bar of soap in your good hand and take hold of your other hand. Your good hand rotates under the palm of the other, which you use as a surface against which to rub the fingers, palm, and back of the good hand. This method will look as though you actually are using two good hands and it gives maximum cleansing results. If you do not have your second hand, soap your good hand and let the thumb perform the cleansing friction using quick strokes over your palm and across the tops and undersides of your fingers.

When this hand and fingernails need further cleaning, use a nail brush or washcloth to assist in this way: rub a cake of soap over your nail brush (use a large brush), then place the brush at a right angle at the back of the

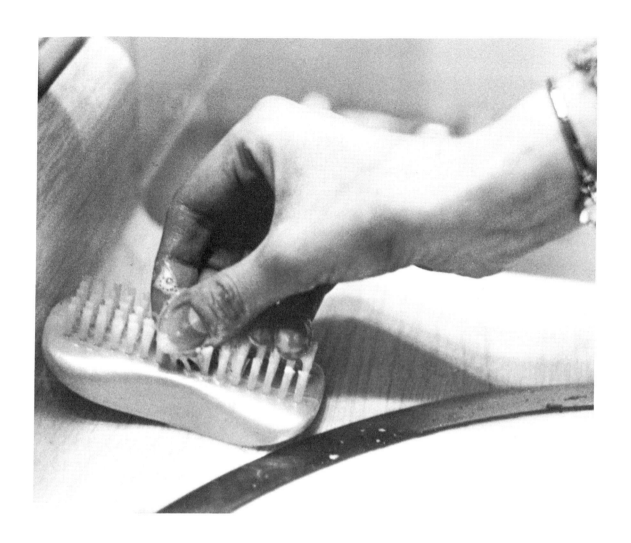

sink basin or on the back ledge of the sink top, to stabilize the brush. Now you can clean all your nails with a few sweeps across the bristles. To attend to the back of your hand, soap a washcloth and lay it at the corner of the sink; rub the back of your hand over it for a good cleaning. Drying your hand is easy even with a paper towel: simply crush the towel in your palm, then lay it down on the sink's edge and turn the back of your good hand over on this to dry it.

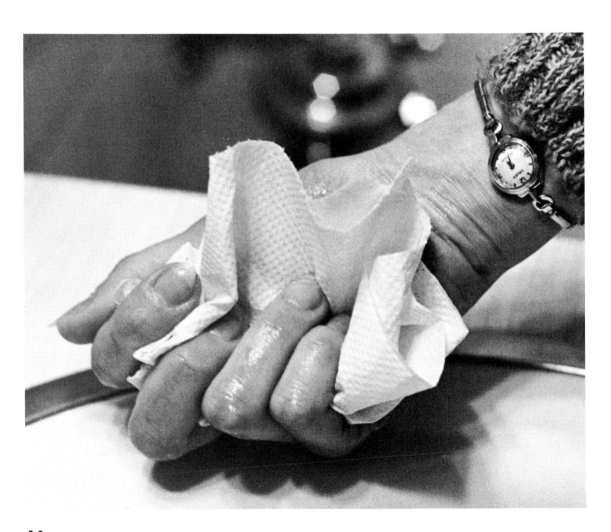

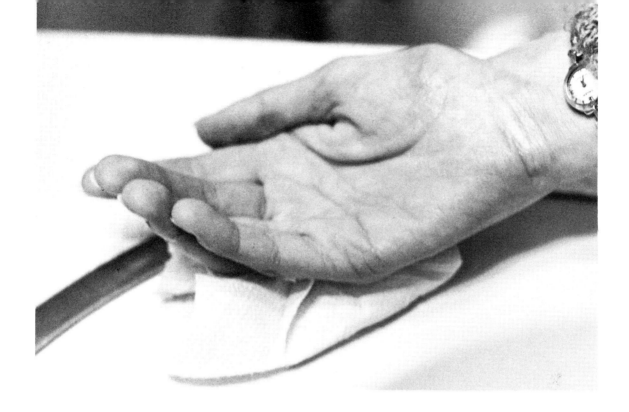

One-handers can perform an almost professional manicure on the good hand; this includes filing or clipping, removing cuticle and old polish, and applying fresh nail polish. To file your nails, use a long emery board; be seated, cross your legs, and place the tip of one end of the emery board between your thighs at the point closest to your knees. It is firm enough now to file one nail at a time without difficulty. Men can clip their nails by

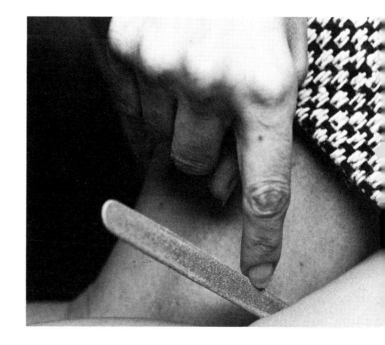

using the pressure of their foot to depress the nail clipper in this way: be seated, place the clipper on the floor and position it under the edge of your shoe. Place your fingernail inside the clipper and step gently on the handle. Trimming the nails of the unusable hand is performed the ordinary way.

bend your fingers in position for painting. Gently guide the brush from cuticle to nail tip. Do not mind how peculiar this may look and feel in the beginning, or how inaccurate your aim the first time you attempt it. (If you are far-sighted, take extra care.) A little practice and this works very well.

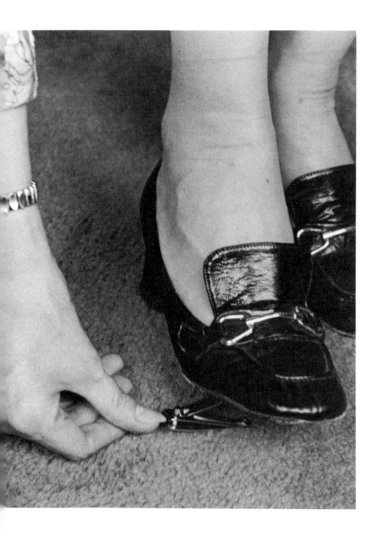

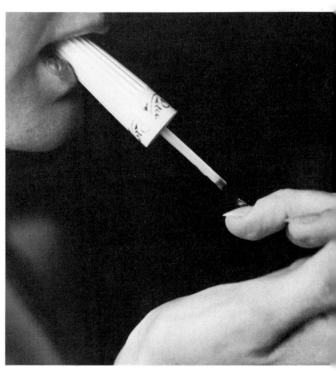

Enamel can be applied to the nails of the good hand. Grip the handle of the brush between your teeth (which perform as your second hand). Hold the brush steady and

Remove nail polish by soaking a cotton pad in the solution; pick the pad up with thumb and index finger and slide the pad back and forth over the four nails with the aid of your thumb, applying circular motions over each nail surface. A cotton pad held under the index or middle finger will remove the polish from your thumb. You can attend to your cuticles the same way.

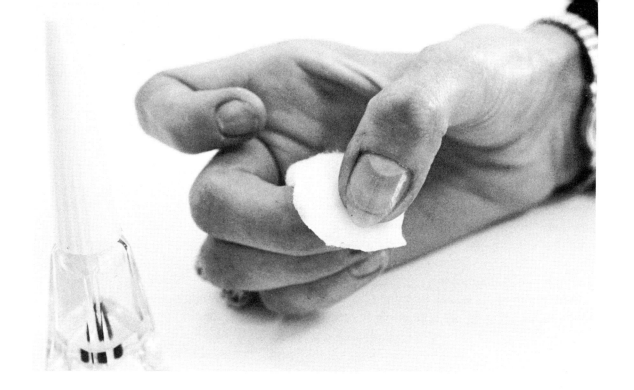

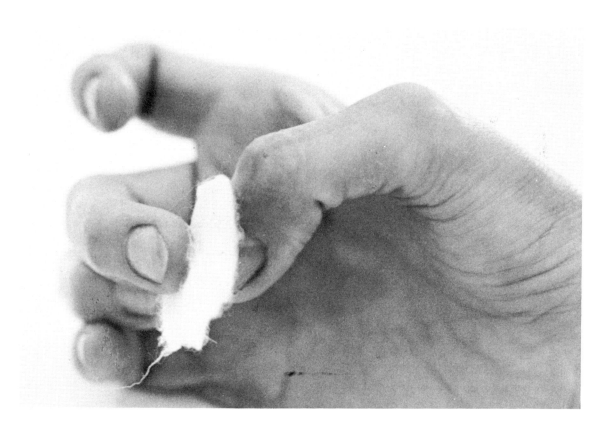

To apply hand lotion use a dispenser bottle, or if you prefer, simply buy small bottles of lotion, which are easier to handle than large ones. If you have your second hand, you can use it to apply the lotion. Be seated and pour a small amount on the back of your nonfunctioning hand and rub your good hand over this. If you do not have your second hand, you may apply lotion this way: pour a small amount of lotion onto your upper knee and rub the front and back of your hand into the lotion. Try to apply as much to the *back* of your good hand, which may tend to be drier because it is harder to reach, as to the palm.

Women will want to lotion the elbow of the good arm to keep it smooth, especially in winter months, and this is done by moving your elbow tip around on the upper knee until the lotion is absorbed.

Each time you use strong cleansing agents such as scouring powders, steel wool, disinfectants, detergents, and the like, slip your hand into a rubber glove for protection. In this way you will keep your hand looking well and working at a peak of efficiency. (That second rubber glove you thought useless can be turned inside out and worn, giving you two "pairs" for the price of one.) If you prefer to work without gloves, keep a bottle of hand lotion at the kitchen sink, in the bathroom, in the nursery and laundry areas, and apply it each time your hand comes out of water. Men are not compelled to such vigilance but women cannot be overfastidious in this area.

During the winter months one-handers must put forth more effort to keep the hand smooth and groomed. Cold weather is particularly harsh to the hand. When it works in combination with household cleansers, the hand often turns red, rough, and raw. It does not look or feel pretty and it may reduce your efficiency. For protection wear good gloves, preferably with a wool lining. Heavier linings such as shearling or fur may interfere with finger dexterity, which we have to avoid. Wear the gloves whether you are outside for five minutes or several hours (see chapter 2, Dressing and Grooming, for the technique of putting gloves on). For greater smoothness in very cold weather use a hand lotion whose label states "for extra dry skin."

If you have a nonfunctioning hand, you will find it imperative to wear a glove on it in winter because the circulation in this arm is poor. Assuming you have sensation in the arm, you will be much more comfortable with the hand gloved and placed in the pocket of your coat. If you have an artificial hand, you may prefer to glove it also to keep your appearance uniform.

During the course of a busy day's activities either at home or on the job one-handers may feel the need to rest the arm once or twice. This can be done simply by taking a few minutes off and raising the arm above your head to a count of ten at those intervals. Occasionally one may experience more than average muscle soreness in the working arm due to a great output of energy. This is only

48

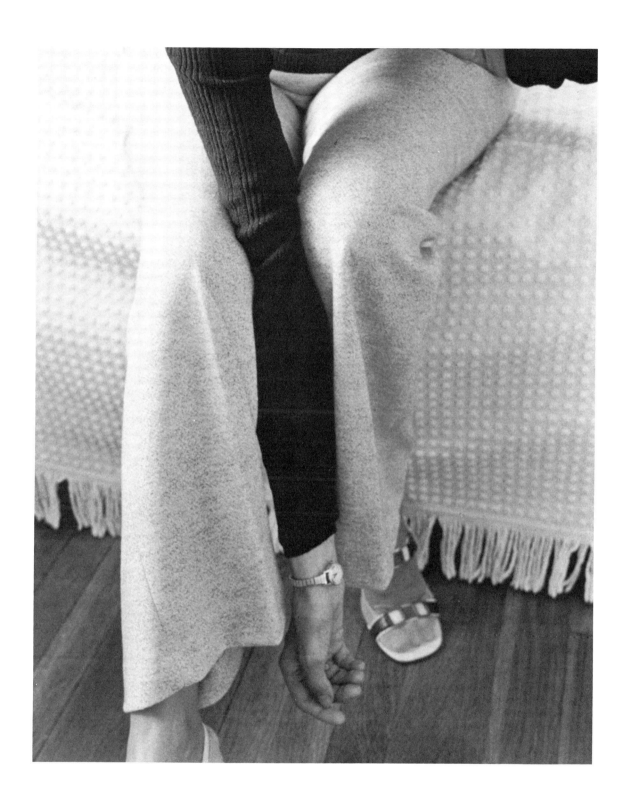

normal, and there is no cause for alarm. A degree of immediate relief is obtained by placing your arm between your knees and then pressing the knees gently to the arm muscles in a kneading fashion. Begin this modified "massage" above your elbow and work down to your fingers. If possible, have someone in your household give your arm a conventional massage, including fingers and shoulder. If one can afford it, a periodic, thorough arm massage by a professional masseuse is recommended.

6

AROUND THE HOUSE

Housekeeping need not be too taxing for the one-handed person. There are lots of shortcuts one can take to maintain pride in one's home or apartment while having fun in keeping it. At the outset a few basic suggestions can be stressed:

1. Take advantage of the spray-can approach to household tasks. Polish the furniture, starch the clothes, preserve furnishings and clothing by spraying. Keep abreast of new products that manufacturers will be packaging in spray cans.

2. Replace dust collectors such as venetian blinds with decorative window shades or with light curtains and/or drapes. In general, keep your furnishings simple; for example, you may have furniture upholstered in heavy-duty vinyl, which keeps the dust and dirt on the surface of the material and is easily cleaned with soap and water.

3. Preserve your upholstered furnishings with a spray fabric protector, preferably when they are new or just cleaned to reduce soil and wear.

4. Buy no-iron curtains, draperies, and slipcovers.

5. Place lots of shelves around, principally in entrance ways, and preferably at waist height. These will hold the thing you need to put down before you are able to carry on in any number of situations. The "shelf" can be a dropleaf counter affixed to the wall in a smaller apartment. Another very helpful item for one-handers is a long table upon which to spread things out and work from.

6. Leave enough space between the bottles, jars, dishes, and canned goods on the shelves of your medicine chest, kitchen cabinets, pantry shelves, china closets, etc., to minimize reaching behind and around objects. Arrange items so that your immediate needs are in front.

7. Line your shelves with plastic or oil-cloth so they can be cleaned with a wipe of the sponge.

8. If possible, acquire furniture that is on casters so you will not have to tug and pull at heavy furniture when you clean. You may prefer to be without heavy furniture made of wrought iron or marble.

9. Keep handy a basket or tray with an over-the-top handle. You will find this very practical for carrying several items as you clean from room to room, thus cutting down on steps. (It goes without saying that buckets and pails must have over-the-top handles for one-handers to manage.)

10. Put up a bulletin board in the kitchen or den and post your notices, clippings, shopping lists, bills, and reminders so you have them at a glance. Shuffling through bits of paper each time you need something can be tedious.

11. Use as many of the magnetic household accessories as you can find, such as pot holders, pens, writing pads, and others. Having these items at hand's reach is desirable.

The foregoing suggestions may benefit almost everyone, but the person who uses one hand will find these, in particular, to be time and energy savers. Some further household tips to help you through your chores are these:

To sweep the floor with one hand, grasp the broom handle under your arm with the top of the handle projecting from the back of your armpit. Your arm is extended halfway down the handle, where your hand grips and

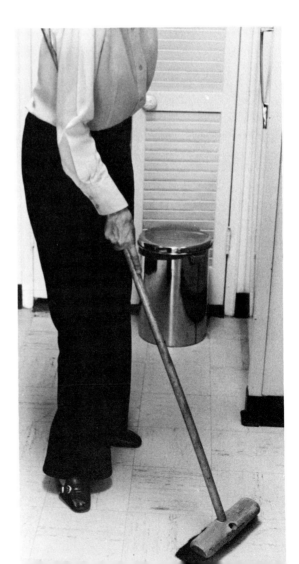

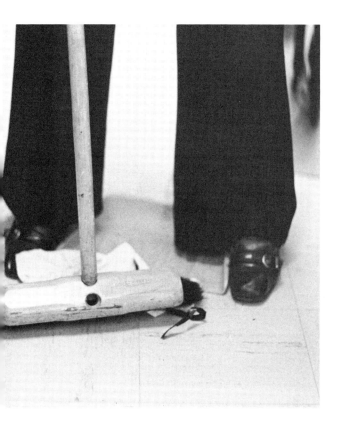

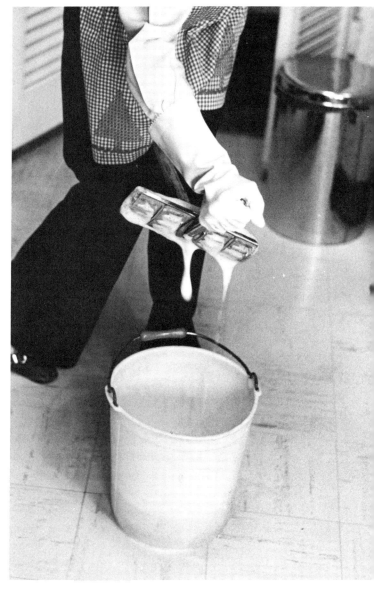

pulls it forward while your elbow provides further support and leverage against your body to effect the sweeping motion. To use the dustpan, set it down flat on the floor and step on both sides of the pan (with either your heels or toes) to secure it.

If you wet-mop your floors, use a sponge mop with its own wringer or a mop of medium-weight strands on a handle of plastic or aluminum. The pail must have an over-the-top handle. To wring the strand mop, first straddle the handle while the mop is still in the bucket; grasp the lowest end of the handle and place it between your knees (the mop head is out of the water and dripping into the pail while most of the handle is protruding behind you). Place your hand underneath the mop strands and squeeze-wring, working your way from the head down to the tips of the mop strands. Left-handers rotate their hand to the right while right-handers wring to the left.

Making beds with one hand is not difficult. The use of contour bottom sheets will

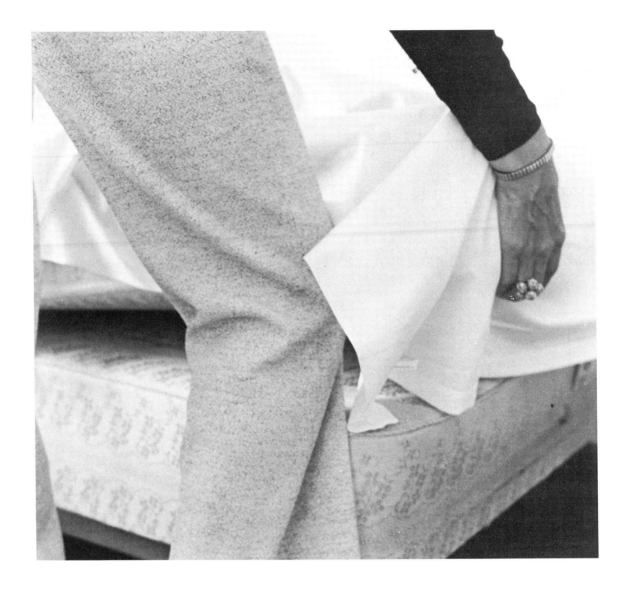

eliminate some mattress lifting. Nylon sheets are light to handle in and out of the wash. If you do not use contour sheets and have a double bed with a heavy mattress, you can use your knees to assist. Lift each corner slightly and insert your knee between the spring and the mattress. This knee support will free your hand to pull the sheet taut and

tuck it under. Make up one side of the bed first, then the other, to save steps.

To put on pillow cases, place the pillow lengthwise perpendicular to the edge of the bed facing you. Spread the case out lengthwise at the pillow's head, open end toward the pillow. Insert one corner, then the other,

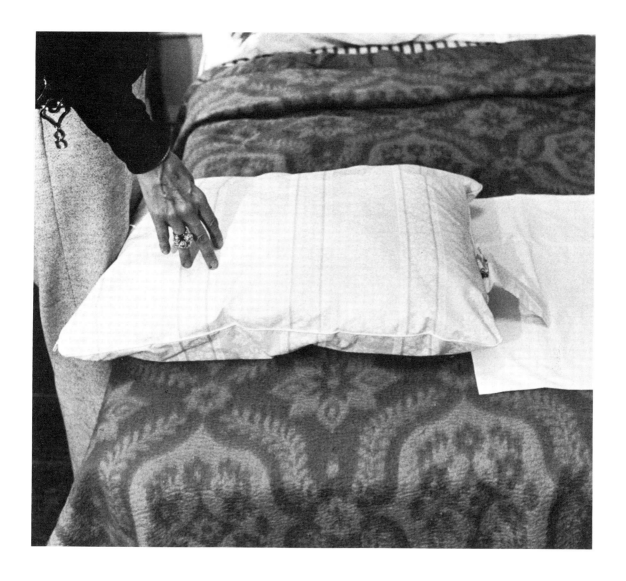

working the slip over the pillow gradually. Work toward your body, supporting the pillow's shorter side at your thighs, and the pillow case goes on easily.

Turning a twin-size mattress with one hand is recommended only for strong individuals. The length of the bed must be against the wall to accomplish this. Slip your hand a quarter of the way under the mattress at the center and pull up. Rest this half-section of mattress against your midsection— take a deep breath!—and insert your whole arm under until your hand reaches the edge of the mattress on the other side. Pull this edge toward you until it rests on its side,

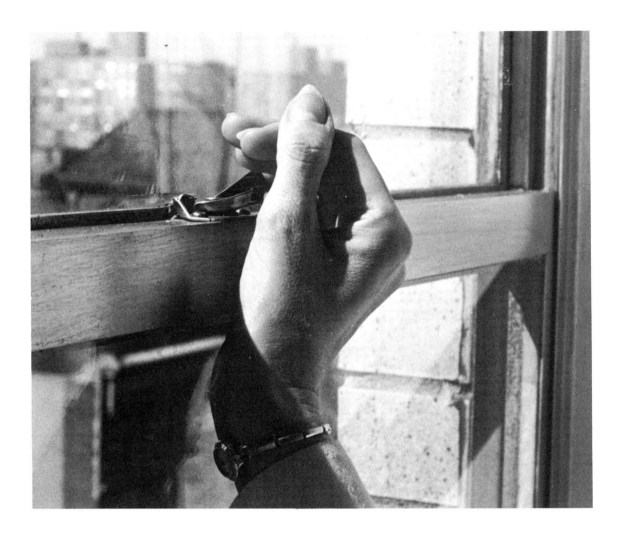

perpendicular to the box spring. With the upper end of the mattress supported against your shoulder, lean forward to topple this section against the wall. Now that it is supported, place your hand at the underside of the mattress at the center and pull it toward you, letting it drop over the box spring where you position it in place. Turning the mattress on a double bed should be done with a second person's help.

For shopping at the food market or the department store, use a shopping bag to carry your bundles home more comfortably. One-handers who walk to the store would do well to own a large shopping cart in which to wheel home heavy groceries and packages.

To open a standard window, position your hand at the center where the upper and lower panes join and push up on the lower window.

Another way is to lift a little on each side of the frame of the lower window until the window is free, then raise it at the center. Washing windows should be no problem. Use a long-handled window brush with a sponge and rubber-tipped wiper at one end.

Use a roller brush to paint walls in the ordinary way. Spray paint is excellent for touch-up and other small paint jobs. To hang wallpaper it is advisable to work with another person just as two-handers do. With today's pre-pasted paper this chore is simplified.

7

IN THE KITCHEN

This chapter is not intended to be a cookbook or menu planner, but simply a guide to the preparation of food. Cooking with one hand is almost as easy as cooking with two hands; if you have the knack, you will cook well in either case.

Ideally, your kitchen should provide a large table or large uncluttered counter space on which to lay out your ingredients and utensils beforehand. It is desirable to have as much as possible at your fingertips before you begin to cook. A practical suggestion is to hang a section of your kitchen wall with pegboard for hanging pots and large utensils. It goes without saying that one-handers should buy pots and pans that have a single handle rather than handles at either side.

One-handers will find that a few kitchen aids are indispensable: a pair of scissors, an electric can opener, an electric knife, poultry shears, a vegetable slicer, and a serving cart.

Use an apron which does not tie but which slips around the waist by means of a plastic band, or buttons or snaps in front, smock style.

Your first task may be the opening of packages, bottles, and cans. Scissors will be helpful with various boxed and bagged items and with packets of luncheon meat and cheeses. Twist off bottle tops while holding the bottle between your knees. To open jars, first tap around the side of the lid using the edge of the kitchen counter, then hold the jar between your knees to steady it while you twist the cap off. Or use a jar opener that clamps over the jar top, adjusting to any size top.

Puncture cans containing liquids either by holding the can between your knees, or for larger cans, by placing the can on a nonskid surface such as a rubber mat, and pressing down hard with a beer-type can opener. The force of puncturing serves to steady the can

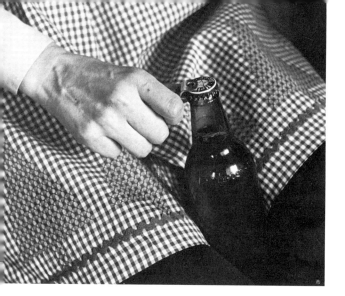

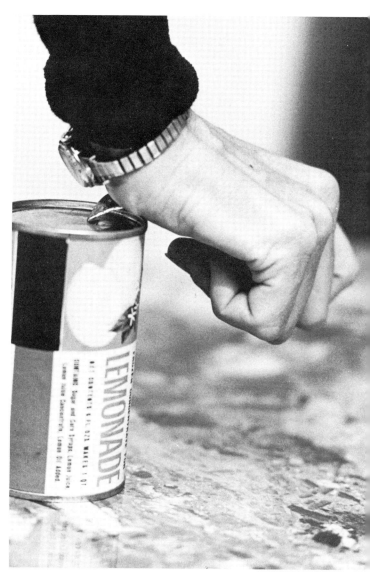

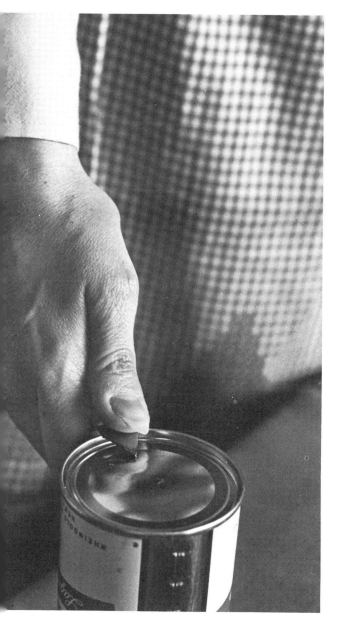

as well. To open smaller cans of liquid such as frozen juice cans, hold the beer-type opener with the sharp tip downward and facing toward your wrist. Hook the opener onto the side of the can furthest from you and press hard on the head of the opener with your palm. Puncture both sides of the can so the liquid pours out more easily.

To open cans containing solid foods, the one-handed person is urged to invest in an electric can opener. This "luxury" item will save a great deal more in time and labor than it will cost in dollars and is a big improvement over the manual wall-type can opener. If, however, you have to use a hand-operated opener, attach it to the wall slightly below the height of your shoulders. Open the clamp and insert the rim of the can by propping the can against your upper chest to hold it steady. Now bring the clamp down hard over the edge of the can, removing yourself from supporting it. Turn the handle to cut through the can, again propping it against your upper chest after you have made a complete cut. Now push the clamp back from the can until you have released it.

Another practical appliance is the electric knife which will enable you to cut large roasts, hams, pork and lamb chops, turkey, and other meats, easily and evenly. One-handers can also use an electric knife to slice melons or other large fruits and for slicing fresh, home-baked or hard-crust unsliced loaves of bread. If you must use a standard cutting knife to slice large fruits, first place the fruit on its side in a horizontal position. Start the cut by placing the knife's point vertically into the center, making a small incision. Withdraw the knife, place the cutting edge across the fruit, and gradually slice through

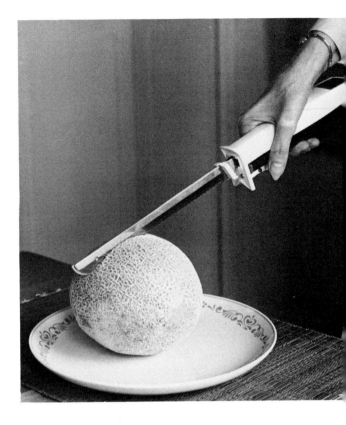

to the bottom. As you can see, this can be done without the fruit's being held by a second hand.

Peeling and slicing fresh vegetables and fruits is something you may have thought would be a problem. Small, round vegetables such as potatoes, onions, and tomatoes, should first be halved and then set down on their "base" to peel or slice them. Potatoes can be boiled first until their skins lift off. For preparing raw fruits and vegetables the one-handed person may use a special wooden cutting board through which aluminum nails project points upward. The board should have suction cups at the corners to steady it. You can press the vegetables down over the nails, thus securing them for peeling, cutting, or scraping. These boards are sometimes found in the housewares section of large department stores. There are various fresh food slicers on the market, manual and electric, which are as easy for one-handers to use as the board. Their primary function is slicing, however, not peeling or scraping.

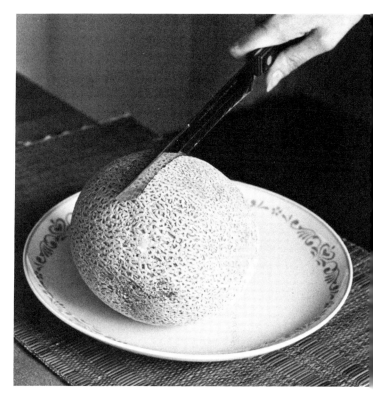

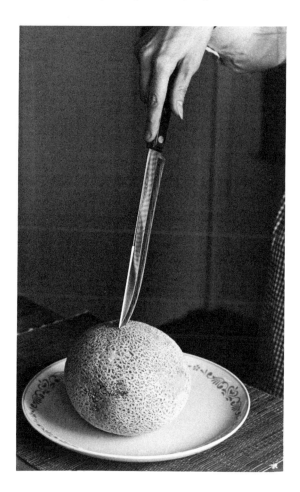

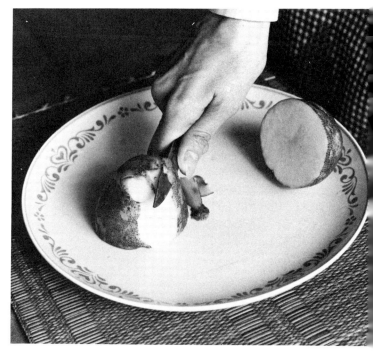

For grating vegetables, stand a four-sided grater on its base and lean forward over the grater's handle with the trunk of your body. With the grater thus steadied under your diaphragm your hand is free to rub the vegetables up and down the grating surface. You can grate two vegetables at once if they are the same size, for example, a carrot and a slice of celery.

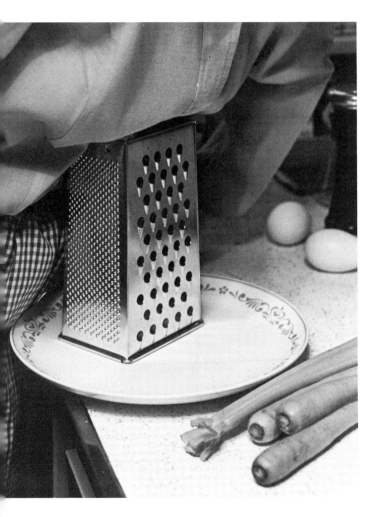

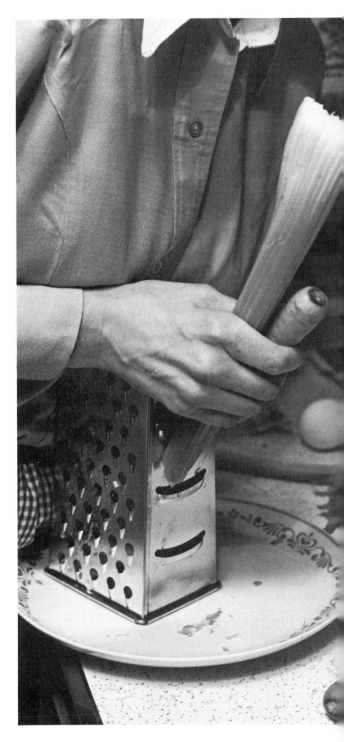

Lovers of fresh garlic will want to have a garlic press. This inexpensive utensil will, with a squeeze of the handle, splice and juice a clove or two of garlic at once, thus saving much time over the slicing method. Other time-savers in the kitchen are the battery-operated pepper mill, the egg slicer, and the baster. The pepper mill might be considered a necessity in more sophisticated cooking. The battery-operated one releases fresh pepper with a touch of the finger. Otherwise, one-handers can use the standard mill by rotating the metal handle with the thumb to the left and right while holding all four fingers around the mill. (The twist-top mill is useless to one-handers.) The egg slicer neatly slices shelled hard boiled eggs for sandwiches or salad. The use of a baster for large roasts and fowls eliminates lifting and tilting heavy pans.

Certain procedures in cooking may at first puzzle the one-handed person. Specifically, these are separating eggs, using a rolling pin, and measuring small amounts of liquid. Most of you have seen a TV chef break an egg with one hand. It amounts to holding the egg over the edge of the bowl and cracking through the center vertically with one quick downward motion of the wrist. With your thumb resting on the edge of the cracked lower shell, in the center, your first three fingers pull the upper half-shell upward, releasing the entire egg. There is a cooking aid on the market that separates egg yolks in a jiffy, although one-handers can do without this device. Just crack the egg on a bowl edge, hold the two shells loosely together, and allow the white to seep out; the yolk is intact.

One-handers can use a rolling pin by placing the good hand over the center of the roller instead of at the handle. (The handles are useless except as a means of picking it up.) Roll the pin back and forth under your palm with short strokes and you will achieve the same effect in rolling the dough as the person who uses both hands.

To measure liquids into a spoon, rest the spoon on a surface and support its handle with a small object before filling. With practice your eye can be trained to measure the correct amount and you can then simply pour

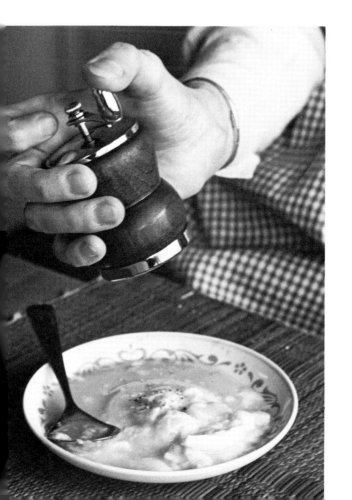

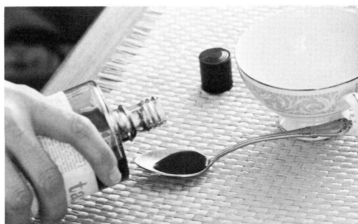

or shake in the ingredient without measuring it. Flat-bottomed measuring spoons are ideal if you can find them.

Here are some further cooking suggestions which may ease the way: stabilize a bowl when hand-beating ingredients by placing it on a large, thin dish sponge or a rubber mat. If you do not have an electric mixer, use the whisk-type beater—it is a natural for one-handers.

Draining foods from a small, light pot is no problem. Pick up the pot and pour the contents into a colander set in the sink. Do not attempt this with a large or heavy pot unless you have the strength for it. Instead, either scoop out the contents with the aid of a small strainer or use a perforated serving spoon, which drains the liquid with each helping.

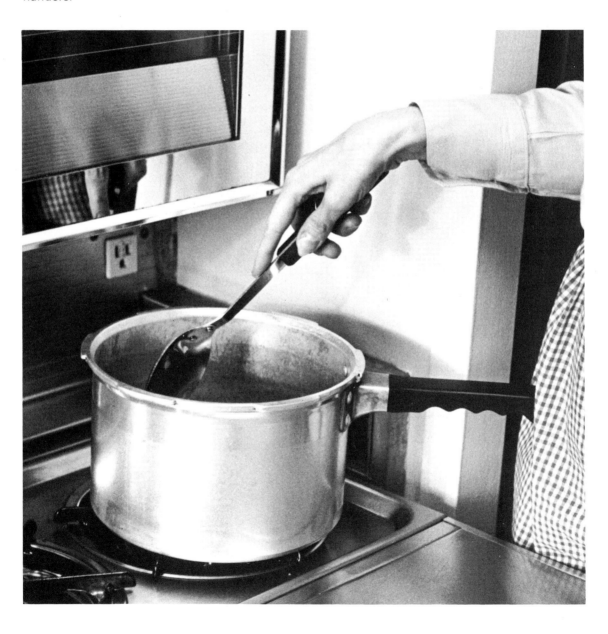

Because you cannot hold the handle of the pot in which food is cooking and stir its contents at the same time, turn the handle so it rests against your hip or midsection, depending on the height of the stove, where it will be secured for stirring. If the pot is heavy and your touch light, this may not be necessary.

A particular convenience for the homes of most one-handed persons is a serving cart on wheels. A cart with a shelf on top and bottom will cut down on countless trips back and forth from kitchen to dining room. You can transport the dishes and food for an entire meal in one operation, whether setting or clearing the table. For home entertaining, the serving cart is almost indispensable as a great time and energy saver. (See chapter 15, Social Occasions.)

The more cleaning chores we can simplify or prevent before they turn into large household tasks, the better. For example, after you have cleaned the refrigerator, place wax paper over the shelves to catch food drippings and change the paper regularly. This avoids scraping and scouring of these parts. The use of aluminum foil for lining the stove and rotisserie is a labor-saving tip. Line kitchen shelves and drawers with self-sticking paper or oil cloth so you merely need to sponge the spots off or to change the paper. The bottoms of sticky jars, cartons, and bottles can be cleaned by rubbing them over a moistened kitchen sponge before putting them on shelves. Of course some real scrubbing is needed from time to time, but this can be kept to a minimum with some forethought. Incidentally, one of the best cleansing agents is common ammonia. When applied full

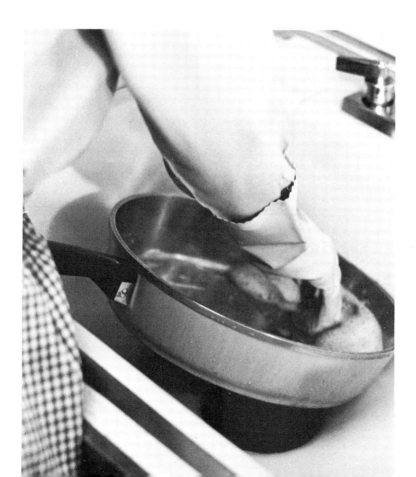

strength it works better than steel wool for cleaning stove tops, the insides of refrigerators, and for removing ingrained stains from kitchen and bathroom appliances, etc.

How do you scour your pots and pans when you cannot hold them still? First, soak the pots immediately after the food is removed. To scour, secure large pots in a back corner of your sink on a rubber mat with the handle facing toward you; if the pot is small, set it in a near corner, handle away. Your scouring strokes on pots in the far corner should be directed away from the body, while the motion should work toward the body on pots in the near corner. The combination of cornering the pot with the use of a sink mat to keep it from sliding (and preventing scratches to the sink) is the formula to keep pots and pans bright and shiny.

Many people prefer to allow dishes to dry in the drain basket rather than wipe them with a dish towel. But if you do use a towel, seat yourself on a kitchen chair or stool and place a dish towel on your lap. Take up another towel and dry dishes individually in your lap. With practice you can dry dishes while standing; take up a plate with the towel and prop the plate against your midsection while you dry it. Let large pans and heavy serving dishes drain dry or towel them dry while they rest in the drainer.

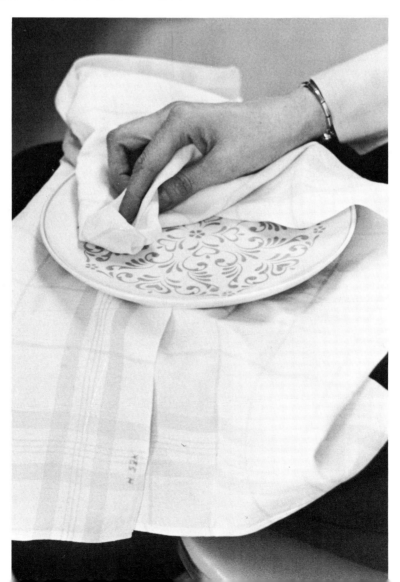

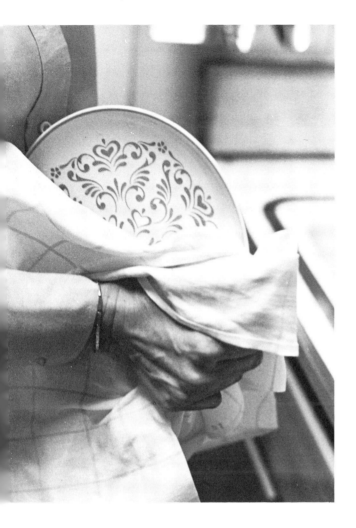

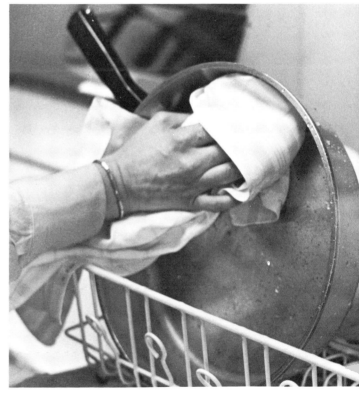

8

WASH AND DRY

In these days of automatic washing machines and dryers you as a one-hander are not going to struggle with the laundering of heavy garments. But to wash lighter garments, such as fine lingerie, which you do not want to wash in the machine, soak them first, then use what should become for you an indispensable household item, the old-fashioned washboard. This is the most effective aid you can have for hand-washing small articles of clothing.

Wringing wet garments can, for the most part, be eliminated, especially if you work in the bathroom or at a large laundry sink and have hooks or rods above the tub or sink from which to hang the dripping garments. Slip an ordinary clothes hanger into the rinse water and place it inside your garment; now raise the hangered garment out of the water, dripping wet, and hang it from the shower curtain rod or over the laundry sink. (It is a good idea to install a spring extension pole over these areas to avoid dripping on the floor.) Shirts, blouses, robes and dresses can be dried this way and even half-slips and skirts can be hung up to drip by slipping the hanger into the waistline and centering it. It is a lot easier to lift clothes out of the water on a hanger than it is to wring them with one hand; women especially find this so. And drip-drying eliminates much ironing. Naturally you will have to wring some articles such as fine curtains or wring when you do not have the facilities to drip the garments from hangers. This is done by doubling the garment in the rinse water and grasping it at the heavier end; now simultaneously squeeze and inch the garment away from you until you have wrung it down to the end.

To hang wash from a clothesline, you can first carry it to the line in an ordinary clothes basket with one hand by supporting one side of the basket against your hip. For big washes, use your food shopping cart as a

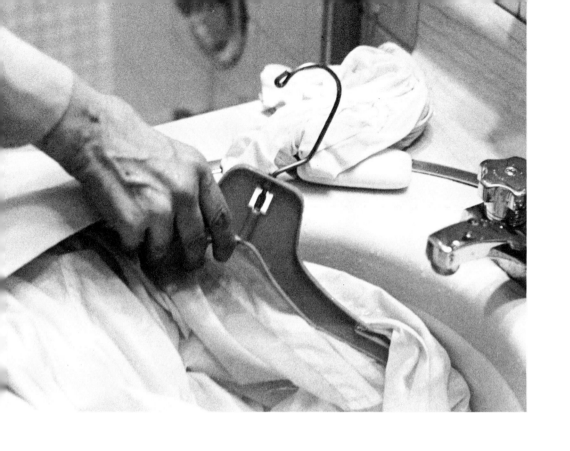

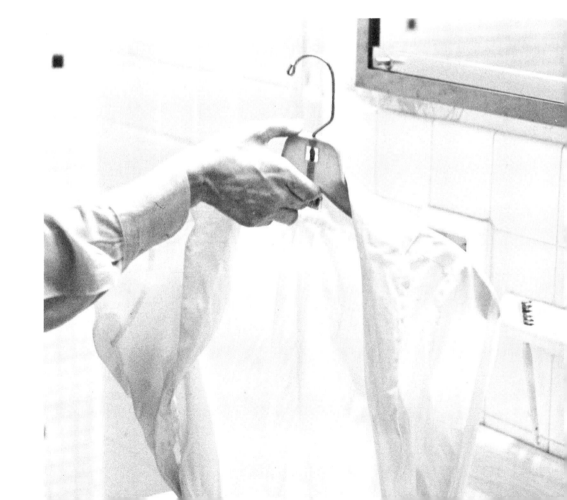

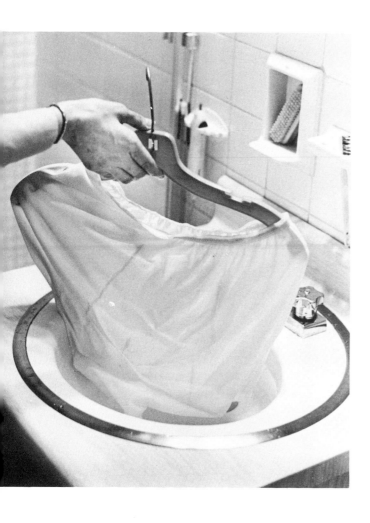

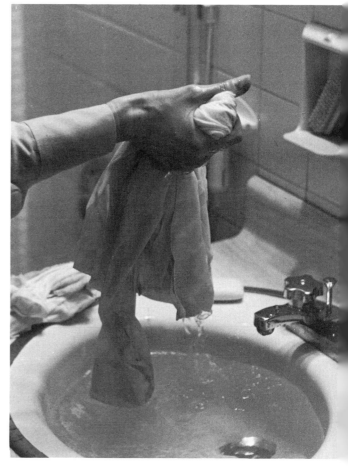

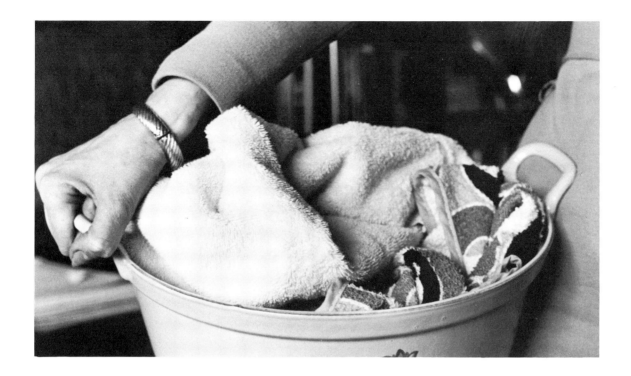

laundry cart; line it with an oversized plastic bag, put your laundry in, and wheel it to the line. You can hand-wring finer garments and put them on hangers to hang on the line; place the regular wash over the line, pin one side, straighten the article, then pin the other end. Use the standard clothespin—not the newer type that requires pinching to open. As you take the wash down, fold it while it is still on the line, that is in a horizontal left-to-right folding position, or the reverse for left-handers. You will see that this method works easiest for you, especially for folding sheets, towels, bedspreads and blankets.

When folding clothes that have come out of the dryer, first spread them out flat on a table or bed. With practice you can use your teeth or your chin as a second "hand" by holding one corner of the garment at either of

these points and the other half in your hand, and then fold corner to corner as two-handers do. Also, you will be surprised how easily your one hand can unscramble the middle section of a sheet, blanket, or bedspread into a precise fold if you first pick up all corners together in your fingers and transfer them to your teeth to hold the article secure.

Ironing with one hand should not be as hard as may be assumed. The difficult part is putting the standard-size board upright. This sometimes requires three hands! When you have to engage chin, elbow, leg, and foot—as well as a strong arm—to erect the ironing board, you will quickly find a corner of your apartment or home where you can leave the board upright. (Your clean board cover may gather dust this way, so protect it with a plastic cover when it is not in use.) As

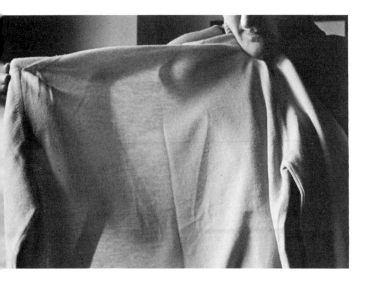

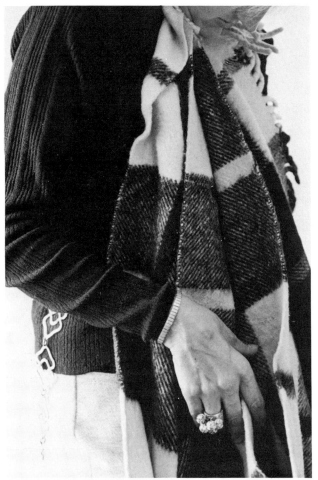

well as can be explained, this is the procedure: tackle the board firmly around its middle, holding one side of the board to your hip. Your hand grips the edge of the board at about the center. If you are left-handed, buttress the lower board against the inside of your left knee for support—right-handers engage the right knee. Now hoist the board straight upward until it is a few inches off the floor. Bend your body forward at almost a 45-degree angle (board in tow!) and depress the lever at the side of the board where your hand is resting. This releases the spring and allows the leg rod to drop into position. If you find this too difficult in the beginning, purchase a small portable ironing board which can be set up on a table. You will not have the large ironing surface which one-handers require, but you may compensate by using a smaller traveling iron. Steam ironing is preferable, of course.

Arrange and smooth out each section of the garment on the board before attempting to iron. Remember the convenience of spray starching!

A tip: one-handers can cut down considerably on washing and ironing summer clothing, in particular, if they will first spray the clothing with a fabric protector on those parts which soil the easiest: the neckband, the cuff and sleeve of the good arm—the seat area and the midriff, hip, and thigh section corresponding to the good arm (see also chapter 2, Dressing and Grooming).

9

NEEDLE AND THREAD

One-handers can master a number of sewing techniques. When we consider that even two-handers use only one hand for the actual sewing, one-handers can accept the practice more readily. The big difference is that it will take you more time. Where two-handers use their other hand to arrange and hold the sewing material, you will use your knees in conjunction with your nonfunctioning hand and/or a paperweight. Sewing is the activity that may require more of your patience than any other. We mention the simple darning of holes in socks, tears in shirts, hems, and sewing on buttons, which we all have need to do at some time or other and which do not require a sewing machine.

To thread a needle, turn it point down into any surface at hand to steady it. This can be a pincushion, the sleeve of your other arm or the lap section of your skirt or trousers. To knot the ends of the thread, place the eye of

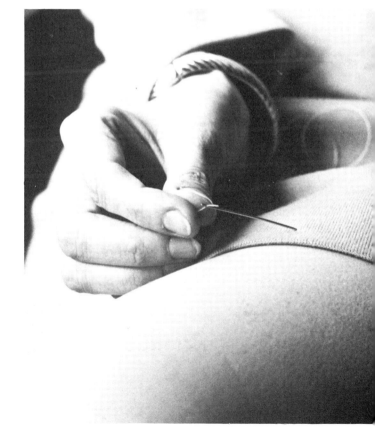

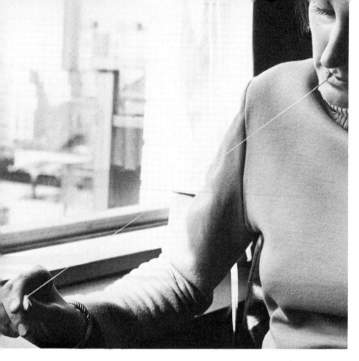

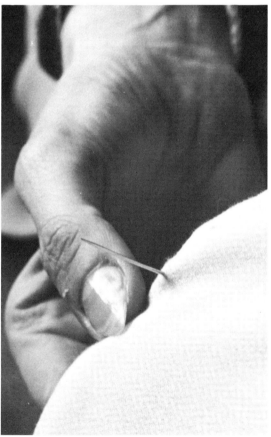

the needle between your teeth to hold it steady. Now you can pull on the thread with your index finger and thumb. Wind the thread around your index finger to knot it in the usual way.

Your knees will serve as your second hand, or anchor, in simple sewing, and your lap provides an adequate work area. The trick is not to catch the needle in the material of your dress or trousers as you sew. To counteract this, use a sheet of tissue paper as a buffer between the garment you are sewing and your lap. If you catch a few stitches, simply tear the tissue away.

To mend a simple tear, place the torn section over one knee and press your other knee to the material to hold it. If your have your other hand, bring it down on the material to secure it more firmly. If you do not have a second arm, work on a table using a heavy paperweight on the garment to secure it. Embroidery loops can also be used for mending tears on larger garments. Secure the sides of the loop horizontally between your knees to hold it and sewing comes easily.

To mend holes in socks, first put the sock on your foot to secure the sewing area; you can tuck a small piece of tissue paper in the opening to prevent the needle's pricking the skin. Or slip a darning egg through the sock and grip this between your knees. Your hand is free to darn the hole.

To sew standard two- or four-hole buttons on easily, work on the knee and hold the surrounding material down by placing your other hand, if you have it, or a paperweight on the garment. First bring your needle under and up through the material at the point

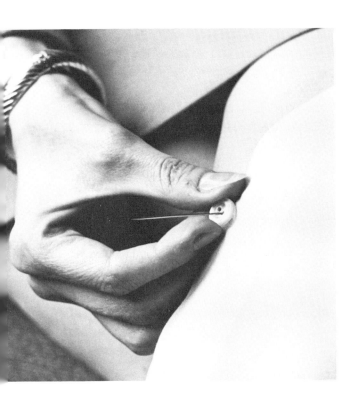

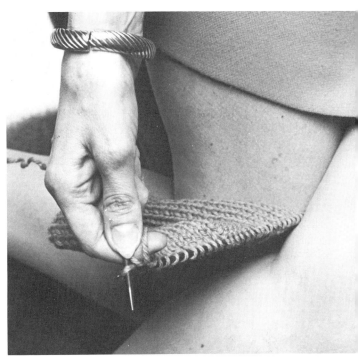

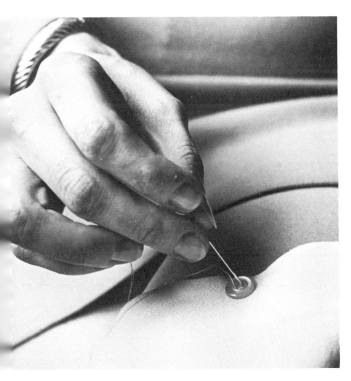

where the button is to be sewn. Now drop the button over the needle and turn the needle point down through a second hole and through the material. The button is now anchored and you can continue the stitch in the ordinary way. As you see, it is not essential to hold on to the button while sewing as two-handers do. Men particularly who might have need to sew on very small shirt buttons, can appreciate this.

For hemming, work from a seated position and guide the hemline across your knees as you sew. Right-handers hem right to left, while left-handers hem in the reverse direction. Your other arm or a paperweight will hold the material somewhat firmly. Or you can hem on a table with a paperweight holding the garment fast. If the material is hard to work with, like silk, wool or a synthetic, it is

75

best to first steam-press the material to the desired width before beginning to hem.

One-handers can enjoy knitting by using longer knitting needles. If you cross your knees you can hold a needle in place where the thighs join and work around this with the other needle held in your hand.

Machine sewing is a wonderful skill to have and you can do beautiful work with one hand. If you like to sew and do not know how to use a sewing machine, by all means take sewing lessons. One-handers can use a sewing machine successfully for making or altering clothes because the actual running is regulated by a foot pedal or an arm wheel while your hand manipulates the material.

10

BABY AND CHILD CARE

The daily activity of caring for babies and young children may be the biggest challenge for one-handed parents or guardians, and you are urged to take advantage of the many child-care aids now available.

Infants can be lifted by a strong arm when it is placed horizontally under the infant's full length with the palm supporting the head and the forearm the outstretched body (the child in a face-up position). If the baby is on his stomach he would be turned over before you attempt this lifting technique. A sitting toddler can be picked up with one hand by approaching him from behind, grasping him around the middle and lifting him with his back toward the front of your body. Young children can be picked up and carried if they are first asked to climb up on a chair, where they are clasped around the waist and held to your midsection. If you have your other or an artificial arm, do not hesitate to grasp it to form an embrace for lifting or carrying children or books or bundles (see also chapter 14, At School). If you are gentle about it, using your other arm this way cannot harm it.

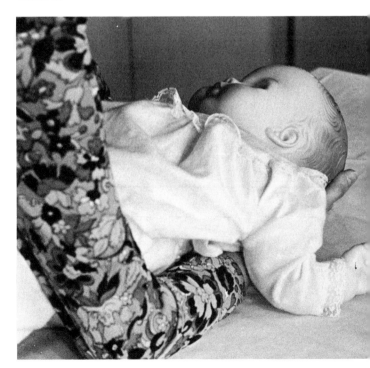

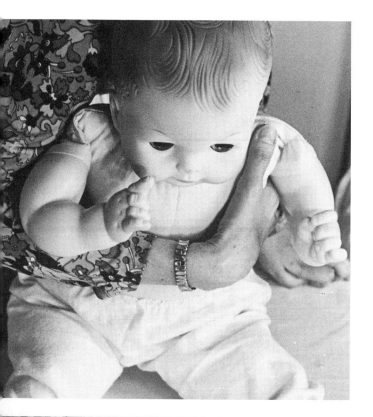

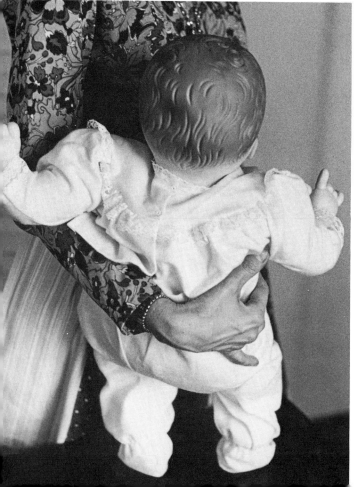

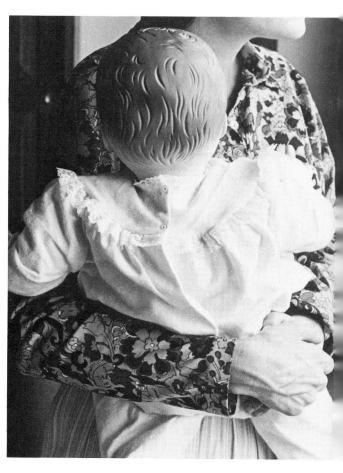

Bathing an infant need not be difficult if you use a reclining plastic stand of the type in which they are carried and often sleep. Make sure the infant is securely strapped in around his middle, then lift baby and stand, anchored against your hip or midsection, into a large, washing pan set in the kitchen sink or a laundry tub. You will not need to be concerned now with holding the baby; your hand is free to bathe it. To wash his back just loosen the strap, turn baby on his stomach, and complete the bath. You can rinse and dry the infant the same way and avoid the unsafe situation of handling a slippery, squirming baby with one hand. Bathing the toddler who can sit up in the tub by himself is easy. Let the water out, rinse him with a spray hose or warm water from a container, then dry him off while he is still in the tub. He can be lifted from the tub by grasping him around the middle from behind. If you need greater assurance that the toddler will not slip from you, you can put on an ordinary cotton or rubber glove before picking him up after the bath.

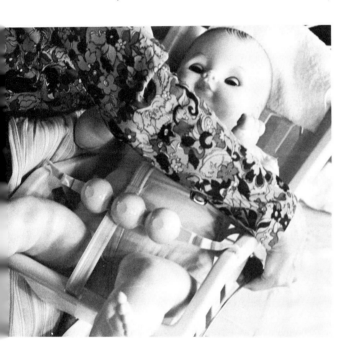

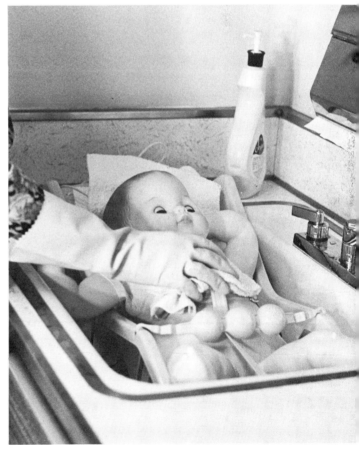

After the toddler or older child's shampoo, use a hair cream or a cream rinse to make combing his hair tearless and easier for you. Further, a natural bristle brush is kinder for unsnarling a youngster's fine hair than a nylon brush.

Babies can be diapered by laying out the diaper beforehand and placing the infant over the point of fold. Use diapers with snaps or the disposable diaper pads which slip into special pants made for the purpose.

Dress the baby on a table or in his crib, not in your lap, because your one arm would be busy holding him still. (How much simpler if little squirmers were able to cooperate when you asked them to put their arms or legs "through here" the way an older child does!) It is strongly urged that one-handers use baby clothes that have zippers, snaps, or elastic openings as these make dressing the infant much simpler. Avoid baby clothes with over-the-head openings. The garment openings for the arms and legs are usually small and tight. You can get around this by slipping all your fingers through the opening, from the outside in, and grasping the baby's hand or foot, gently easing it through. The procedure with older children is to let them dress themselves by showing them where to put their arms and legs while holding that portion of the garment in position for them.

Putting on the baby's socks and shoes may seem difficult, or impossible, in the beginning. Begin by positioning the baby in his crib or on a table so his back is propped up against your midsection. Now at least he is set up to help with an occasional "kick," sure to come from him. To tie shoelaces on the baby's foot, see chapter 2, Dressing and Grooming. (Until the baby walks use soft slipper-shoes that zipper on.) You can tie an older child's shoelaces by sitting down and having him stand between your knees, with his back facing you, your legs skirting his. Now with his foot in the exact position as yours is for your own shoe tying, you will have no trouble tying his the same way.

To give a bottle to an infant while he is cradled in your arm, first be seated and cross your legs. This will raise the baby slightly. Prop the baby against the upper part of either your good arm or your nonfunctioning arm, which provides a perfectly secure "cushion" for him and will not be harmful to your arm. Cradling him firmly against your chest and arm, hold the bottle to his mouth. Secured in a high chair or carrier, he can be spoon-fed with no difficulty.

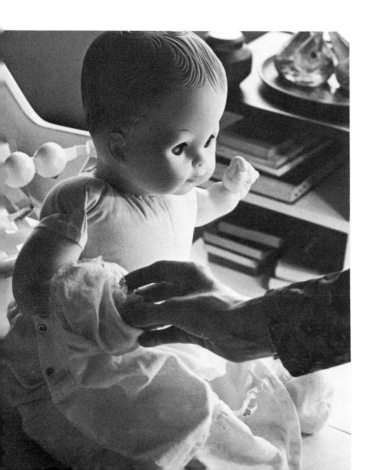

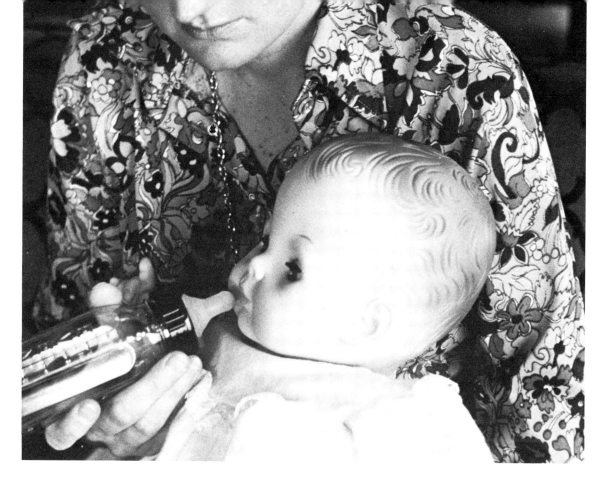

You will occasionally have to carry the infant with you while you shop, travel, or go on errands, but obviously you cannot carry him for long periods in your arm (or arms). A great boon to parents with one hand is the baby carrier that straps the baby securely to your upper back or chest, piggy-back style, and leaves your hand free for your activity. These carriers are popular with two-handed parents now and should be standard equipment for one-handers. Another "indispensable" for you is the baby harness and leash. With the baby secure inside the harness, the leash is fastened to a belt around your waist. The few yards of leash enable the child to toddle along safely with you—in the house, in the back yard, or in the supermarket.

11

DINING OUT

You can handle most things on the menu during the course of a meal without calling attention to the fact that you are using one hand. Many people ordinarily dine with one hand in the lap.

To pull yourself smoothly to the table, try this: as you seat yourself, take hold of the side of the chair adjacent to your good arm and engage the foot that is opposite to this arm around the front chair leg at the side of that same foot; now move yourself and the chair forward in one or two movements. A left-hander will engage his right foot and the right-hander his left foot. In this way your foot deftly takes the place of a second hand.

Cutting meat is the biggest obstacle at table. A smaller one is buttering bread. Of course you will be less concerned with strict table etiquette when eating at home than you will be at a formal dinner or on a date (see chapter 15, Social Occasions).

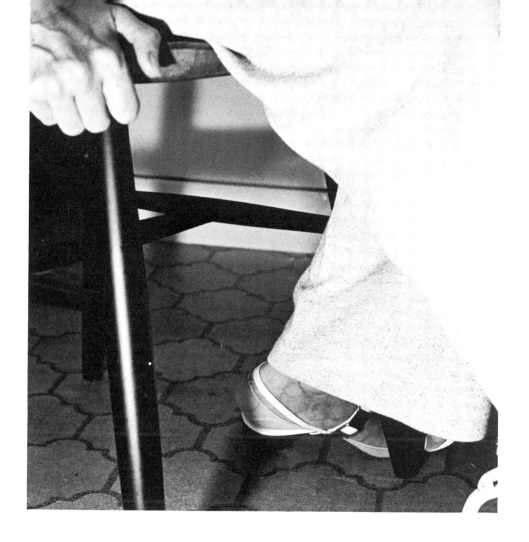

When dining out you may prefer to order an entree that does not require much cutting. You can eat chopped steak, meat loaf, boned chicken, chicken livers, and fish with the aid of a fork alone. With a little practice the one-hander can handle cuts that are firmer, such as roast pork or braised beef ribs. In general, beef—steak and thickly sliced roast beef—are difficult to manage.

For one-handers the key is to start with an extra-sharp knife. But because many restaurants do not provide them, you will either have to ask the waiter for a steak knife or carry your own with you, with blade protected in tinfoil.

For thick cuts, place the point of the knife at the meat's center, aligning the knife with the grain for easier carving. Sink the knife

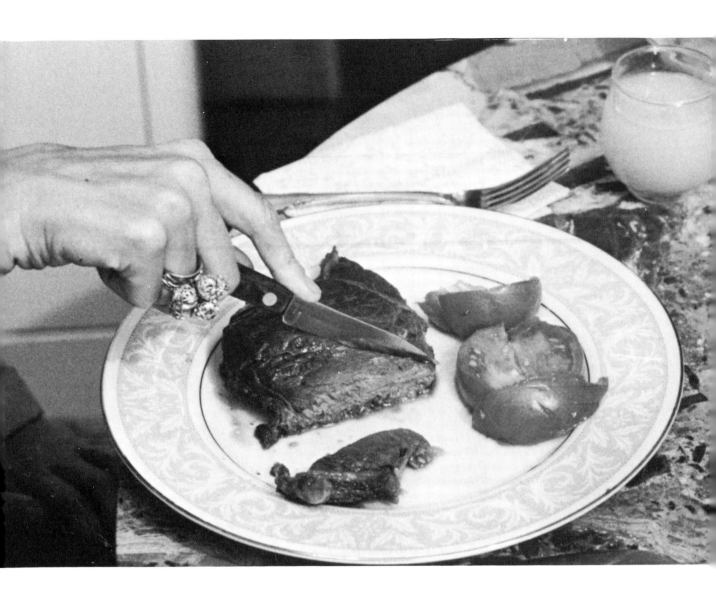

down as hard as you can; now raise the knife out and repeat the step. Of course you work toward the edge of the plate. This in-and-out motion works easiest for one-handers because it prevents the meat from sliding, which the sawing method used by two-handers would cause. As you cut each slice, keep turning your plate so you always work toward your body. You might cut a few pieces at a time to allow for a respite and to keep the meat from getting cold.

As a general rule, recent one-handers with a liking for seafood will feel more comfortable when dining out, particularly in the beginning, if they order such dishes as filleted fish, lobster newburgh and crabmeat thermidore, rather than whole lobsters. At home, of course, one is free to grapple with shellfish any way one chooses. Managing oysters and clams on the half-shell requires some practice. First secure the shell against the thumb of your good hand to steady it. With the head of the fork inverted in the meat's center and in a firm grip under the index and middle fingers, tug the fish toward you (your thumb, that is) in one scoop to free it.

One-handers can manage lobster tails that have been split. A strong hand can "roll" the meat loose this way: poke the last two prongs of your fork into the meat and press down hard with it on the shell to keep the shell from sliding; now roll the fish either to the right or left to free it of the shell.

Jumbo cooked shrimp in the shell can be cut with a knife and often a fork. If cut into small pieces, shell and all can be taken into the mouth where fingers aid in removing the meat. This comes more naturally in the privacy of home. There you can take up the whole cooked shrimp in hand and pry the meat out by mouth.

When pheasant, hare, turkey, hen, or other fowl or limbs therefrom are to be eaten, use your fork to remove most of the meat. Pick up the smaller bones in your fingers to finish off.

The only difficulty you may have with a salad, unless the lettuce is very crisp, is trying to cut the lettuce with a fork. Wilted or oiled lettuce responds better to a knife.

When bread and rolls are served, break them first into sections before buttering them. You can either quarter soft bread with a knife or pull the corners off with one hand. Harder bread, like pumpernickel or rye and soft rolls can be handled like this: pick up the slice and hold it with the last three fingers against the heel of your hand. With your index finger and thumb pull the other half away; work your way down the slice until you have severed the bottom crust. Small, hard rolls should first be broken in your hand over your plate. With one end gripped under your last three fingers, pull the top end apart with your thumb and index finger. Break up the roll a section at a time. When dining out, butter the sections of bread on the bread plate. The dish will tilt some but not uncomfortably so. At home you can place the bread right at the side of your plate on a napkin and butter it on the table.

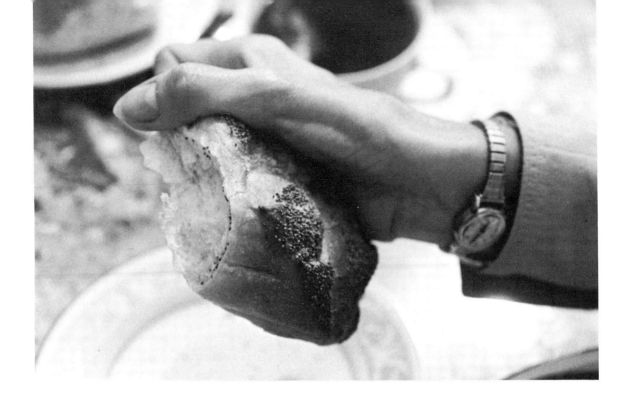

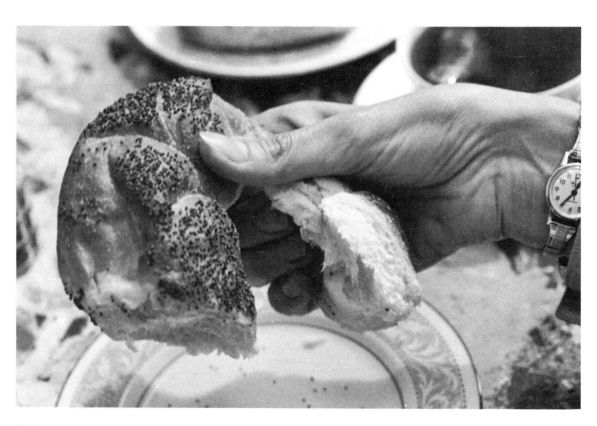

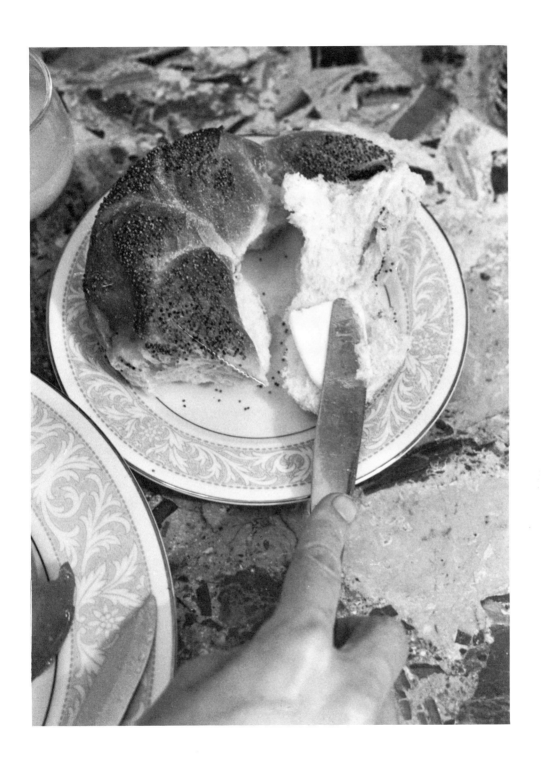

Eating large hamburgers and three-decker sandwiches is a graceless feat for most. The fastidious one-hander may want to avoid them altogether in public.

Other food-handling problems you may encounter when dining out are sectioning fresh grapefruit halves and peeling hot soft-boiled eggs. (At home, when eating fresh grapefruit that is not sectioned, you can hold half of this fruit between your knees to steady it. Sectioning it then is easy.) When a grape-fruit half is served you as appetizer or dessert at a dinner, unless a serrated grapefruit spoon accompanies the fruit, do not attempt to handle it, but sit that course out. One-handers cannot manage grapefruit with an ordinary teaspoon without a struggle. If a serrated spoon is at your disposal you may be able to handle unsectioned grapefruit by positioning the base of your palm at the fruit's edge to hold it steady while your fingers work the spoon into the fruit. Recent one-handers

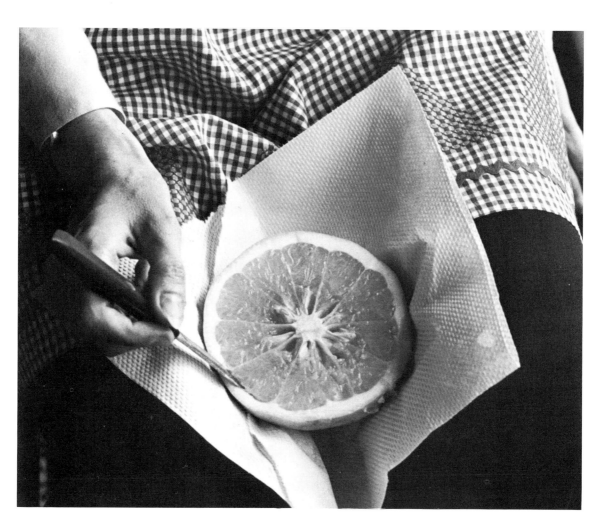

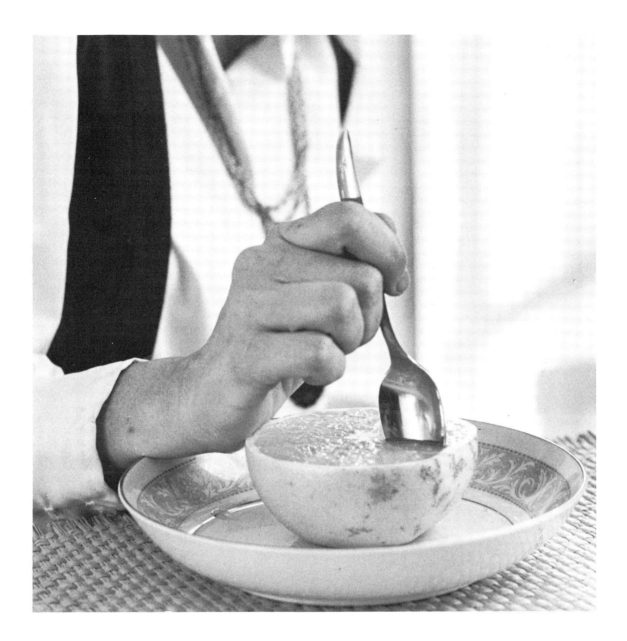

must work up more finger dexterity for this. Hot soft-boiled eggs in the shell can be manuevered in an egg cup, an item as indispensable for one-handers as the scrubbing board or the electric can opener. An egg cup holds the soft-boiled egg secure and prevents fingers from getting burned, while it keeps the egg warm for eating. By itself the egg cup takes the place of a second hand. Use it this way: remove the egg from the hot water and place it, tip upward, in the cup. Tap a small circle around its top with the spoon and lift

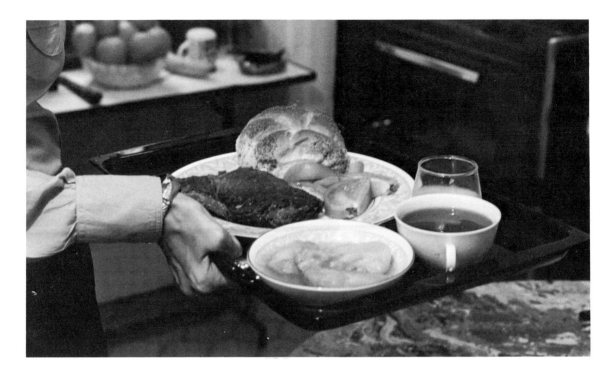

this "cap" free. Now gently spoon your way down through the yolk; the shell remains intact. This is perhaps the cleanest way to eat soft-boiled eggs.

If you occasionally eat in a cafeteria, the secret to carrying a dish-laden tray with one hand is first to start with a strong arm, and second to eliminate all unnecessary plates from the tray. With practice, the stout-hearted can carry food trays with aplomb in this manner: place your main dish, the heaviest, at the bottom edge of the tray and center it. If you are right-handed, place salad dish, milk glass or coffee cup, and small dessert dish at the right side of the tray; left-handers arrange them on the left side. Leave off the bread plate, the saucer, and the under dishes, as these add needless weight. The bread goes on the food plate and you can go back for the saucer if you must. Now get a good grasp in the center at the tray's edge to lift it up. It is to be expected that you will wobble a bit in the beginning, but repeated tray carrying will strengthen your hand and arm and allow you to carry the tray a short distance safely.

12

IN TRANSIT

You can have full confidence in your ability to get around freely if you remember the cardinal rule for one-handers: *travel light.* This holds equally for an excursion around the world or a walk in the neighborhood. Have your fare or ticket in hand, where possible, or in a pocket for quick removal (see chapters 1 and 4, Everyday and Fashion-Wise).

Women and girls should purchase handbags with generous handles, or better, buy shoulder-strap bags, which are ideal for one-handers because they leave the good hand free. Handbags with zipper or snap openings on top are easier to handle than envelope-type purses. Clutch bags are best left for those occasions when you have an escort to open doors and generally help you navigate.

Cameras and binoculars with sturdy straps can be carried over the shoulder or around the neck. In traveling, particularly, will one-handers feel most secure if the good hand is kept free to maneuver with.

Umbrellas can be manageable. Naturally, the push-button type is easier for one-handers. In fact, this is a marvelous invention for everyone, but the one-hander (man, woman, or youngster) should find it indispensable. Purchase one with a curved handle rather than a straight or chain handle so that you can hook it over the back of a chair or other resting place when you need to free your hand quickly.

If you use a standard umbrella, an easy way to open it is to hold it in a horizontal position, place its tip up against a nearby building, press in on the release lever, and push forward until the umbrella locks into place.

In choosing luggage, you will find that fabric or vinyl bags are most practical for one-

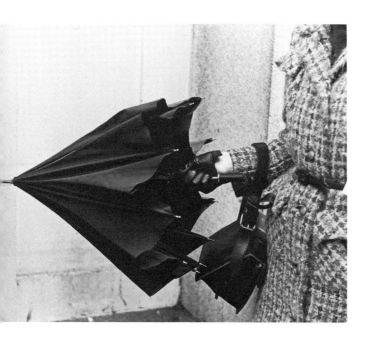 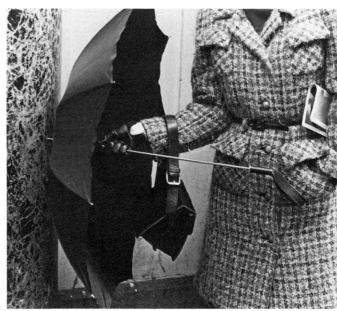

handers. The obvious advantage is their light-
ness, and a zipper opening top is far simpler
to handle than the usual side locks on standard luggage. (A practical packing tip is to slip
clothes hangers into shirts, blouses, dresses,
etc., as you pack them; then you can lift them
out, already hanging, when you have reached
your destination. Of course this requires
larger rectangular luggage.)

If you have a heavy piece of luggage to
transport, you may find it worthwhile to invest in a portable luggage carrier on wheels.
One lightweight model has a slim aluminum
rod and small wheel base. Upon arrival at
train or plane you unbuckle a strap to release
the luggage and the rod slides down for easy
carrying. Luggage carriers are a boon to
travelers in general, but are especially practical for one-handers on the go.

13

FROM NINE TO FIVE

One-handers are capable of performing all the duties called for in a business office. The only difference is that these tasks may take you slightly longer than your colleagues to perform.

When you are opening mail, your chair should be pulled in close to the edge of the desk. You can place a piece of mail between the desk edge and your midsection to secure it, then slit the envelope open with your thumb or a letter opener. Mail can also be held firm for opening by placing it between your knees or inserting it in the crack of a closed desk drawer, with flap section out, then slitting the envelope open. But life gets simpler all the time; many busy offices now use electric letter openers.

If your office does not have an electric pencil sharpener, you can use the standard wall type. If it is placed low on the wall, hold the pencil in the sharpener by pressing your hip or upper thigh against the pencil's end. If

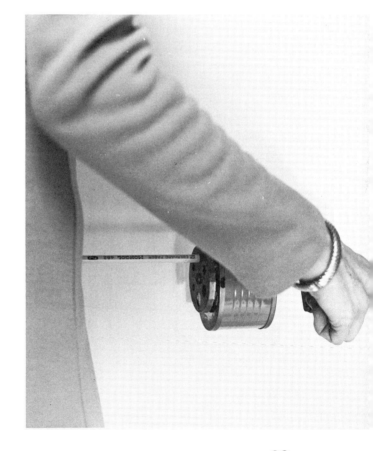

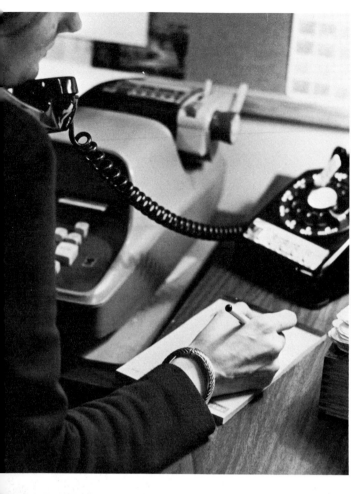

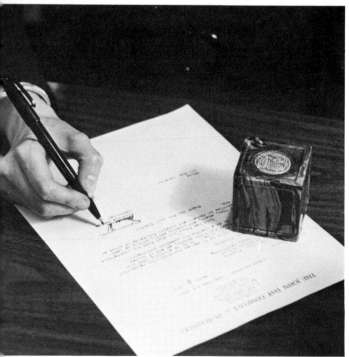

you apply sufficient pressure, the pencil should not spin loosely in the sharpener and you can turn the handle with your good hand. If the sharpener is placed fairly high on the wall you can use your upper chest to hold the pencil in position. Sometimes a small pencil will spin, and your one recourse then is to grip it between your teeth to secure it for sharpening. However, you may not want to do this in anyone's presence!

For signing correspondence use a ballpoint instead of a fountain pen simply to save the small effort of screwing the cap on and off. To loosen the cap of a fountain pen, hold the pen between your knees, or in your palm under the last three fingers and unscrew the top with your thumb and index fingers.

Writing surfaces can be held securely with a paperweight or your nonfunctioning arm. Simply place it by means of your good arm in the center of the paper or at the upper edge of an envelope you wish to address by hand.

When taking phone calls, you may want to use a telephone shoulder hook which fits over the receiver and rests on your shoulder, freeing your hand to write down messages. The more agile can cradle the receiver at the neck between shoulder and jaw, although this requires some practice for long sessions of taking down notes over the telephone.

Typing with one hand is not as prohibitive as it may at first appear. One-handers can accurately type from 45 to 55 words or more a minute on an electric typewriter and even find it pleasurable.

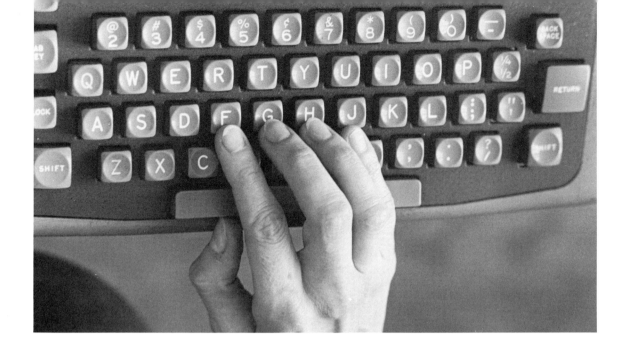

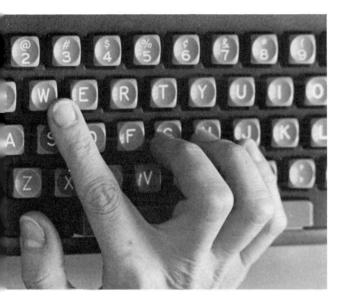

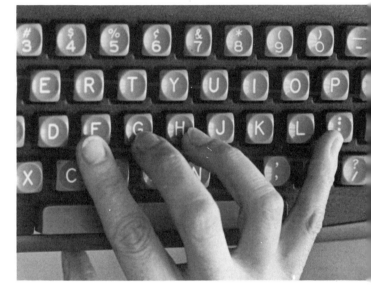

Using an electric typewriter minimizes the strain on your arm and shoulder, particularly during long sessions of typewriting. The technique is as follows: center your four fingers on the base or guide keys of F-G-H-J. The right-hander's index finger controls the left keyboard, first four keys of each row, and the little finger controls the last five keys of each row on the right of the board. The thumb, of course, rests on the space bar. The left-hander's index finger controls the first four keys of each row on the right keyboard and the little finger controls the last five keys of each row at the left of the keyboard. The two middle fingers move the least. They rest over keys G-H and are used for the T-Y on the upper and B-N on the lower rows. The hand leaves the keyboard to depress the shift-lock key for capitals and returns to the guide keys.

Right-handers may shift for capitals on the right side of the board by pressing the shift key with the little finger and striking the desired letter with the index finger. To type capitals on the left side of the board, depress the shift lock with the middle finger and move the fingers back to the guide keys. Left-handers reverse the technique.

When filing heavy materials, mark your place in the file drawer by picking out a folder at the correct filing spot and tilting it slightly on its side to hold it up as your marker. File your material in front of that marker. If you want to read a paper from the file that you expect to refile immediately, make use of your other arm, if you have it, by bringing it up with your good arm to keep your place in the file. This method works best if the file material is at waist level.

To remove a group of folders or very bulky material from the file cabinet, slip your hand

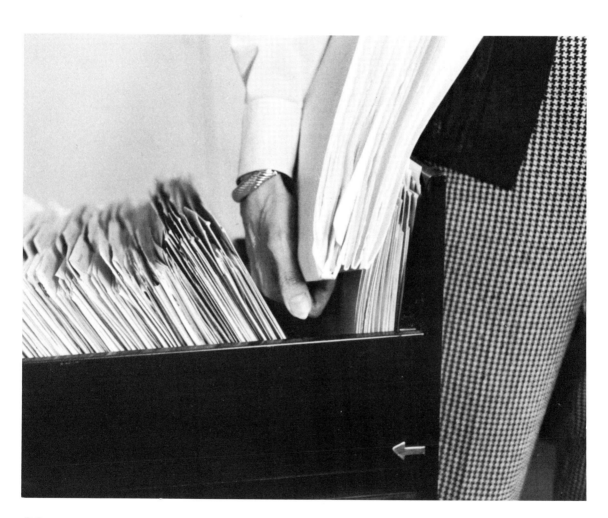

down and under the folders and bring them out.

Index cards can be filed quickly by holding the corner of the card between thumb and index finger. Locate your filing place with your middle finger and separate the cards with the fourth finger. Then drop the card into place.

Affixing paper clips, staples, and rubber bands does not require a special technique but perhaps more time and care to achieve neatness. The recent one-hander, with patience, will acquire efficiency in this.

A clothing tip for the office worker who wears long sleeves: wear a plastic sleeve protector on the good arm, or on both if you have the second arm, to keep the sleeves and cuffs from wearing and soiling quickly.

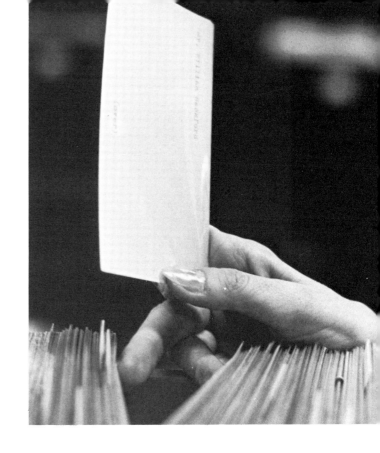

14

AT SCHOOL

From junior high school through college and adult education courses you will be carrying heavy books with your good arm, or cradled between your two arms, as explained below. During the high school years it is customary to carry around books for a full day's course load. And you will sometimes have to negotiate closed doors with the same hand with which you carry your books.

You may find it simpler to use a book bag to carry your books, but this does entail packing and unpacking books between classes, which can be bothersome. It is often simpler to scoop the books up from your desk with your good arm or "arms" and "hug" them to your chest before you dash out the door (a prerequisite for this, of course, is a second arm). If you have the arm, use it by all means; you cannot do harm to yourself if you are gentle. It can be done this way: lock your good hand at the wrist or forearm of your nonfunctioning one to hold the books securely inside both arms. This carrying position looks natural and it is comfortable, more so than carrying many books in one arm. However, if you do not have your second arm and must carry many books at once, you will be more comfortable with a book bag. Incidentally, your good arm will gain in strength during your book-carrying school years!

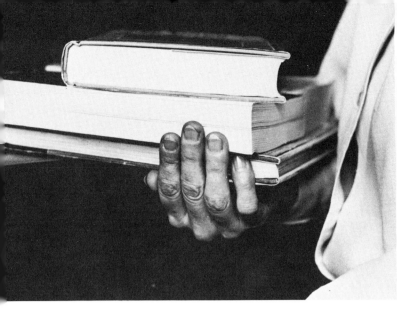

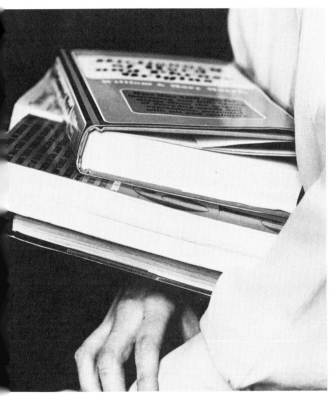

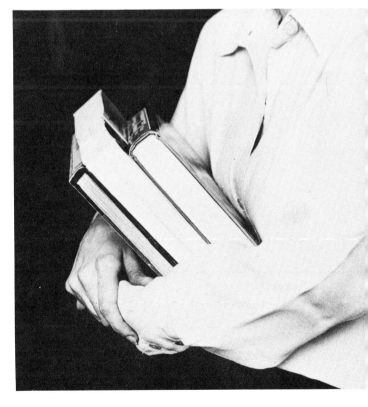

99

When confronting a closed classroom door that opens inward, with your arms loaded with books, you must disengage your thumb and first two fingers from your other arm in order to turn the doorknob. Push the door in slightly with your knee to enter and close the door by nudging it with your elbow. If the door opens outward, firmly grip the doorknob, back up a step or two as you open it slightly, and slip your toe in the door to pull it open. Naturally, it is easier for recent one-handed students to open and close classroom doors with their books in a bag rather than held in an arm or both arms. After a while you will acquire speed and dexterity using your foot as a door opener. Again, if you do not have your other arm, you will find a book bag more practical.

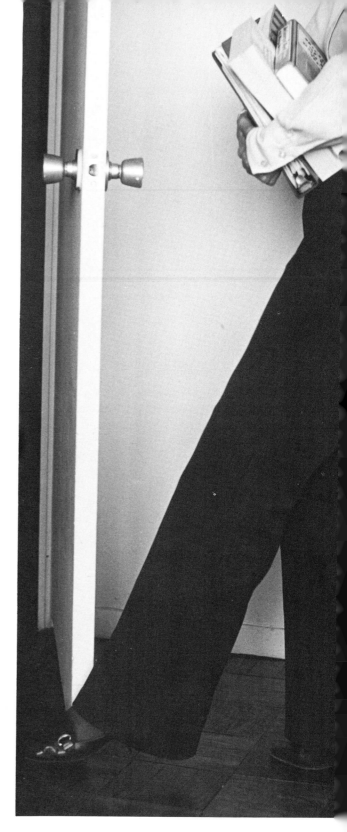

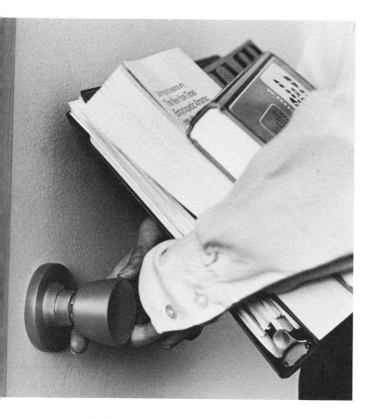

Spiral-bound notebooks are easier to write in than ones with regular bindings because they allow the pages to lie flat. You may use a text book as a paperweight for writing on loose paper. If you have your other arm this will serve as your paperweight; place it with your good arm over the center of the paper to steady it.

For studying at home you may find a bookstand helpful for holding your books upright; this will also free your hand to take notes.

Your may want to use pencils for your class work, but the problem of keeping them sharpened comes up. Best to sharpen a supply of them at home or use a retractable lead pencil.

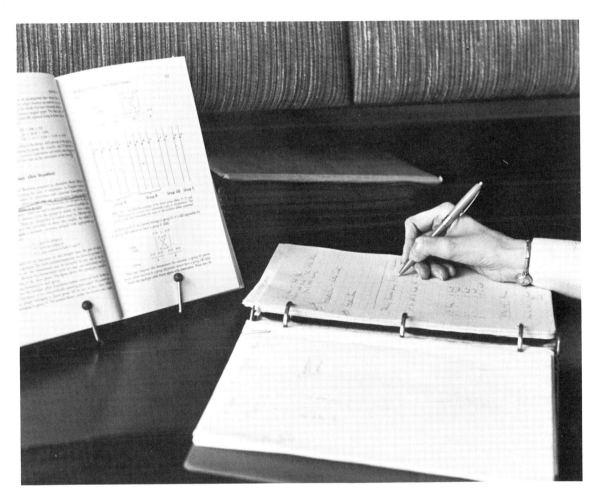

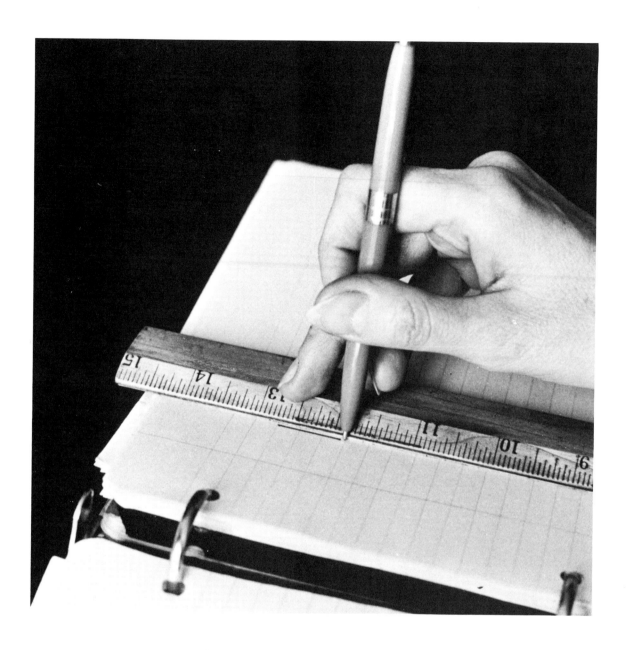

Using a small ruler with one hand to underscore words or sentences will be a little difficult at first until you have built up finger dexterity. Arrange the ruler and material so that you draw on a vertical line instead of on the horizontal, as two-handers do. Hold the ruler firmly under your last three fingers and draw the line, a small section at a time, with your thumb and index finger until you have reached the end. You can work from top to bottom or the reverse, whichever comes easier. If you use a long enough ruler and have your other arm, you can underscore in the usual horizontal way by bringing the elbow of this arm onto one end of the ruler and bearing down on it while you make the line. For special work at home or office, that requires a great deal of repeated measuring or line drawing, you can use a "paperweight" ruler; these are heavy enough to allow you to rule without holding the ruler, which will be less fatiguing.

A clothing tip for the student who wears long sleeves: wear a plastic sleeve protector on the good arm, or on both if you have the second arm, to keep your sleeves and cuffs from wearing and soiling.

15

SOCIAL OCCASIONS

Since one-handers will mix socially in a two-handed world, a few suggestions may be helpful.

Hand shaking, though no problem for right-handers, may seem awkward to the recent left-hander. However, left-handers need not hesitate before shaking hands. It is surprising how quickly people respond to an extended left hand, adjusting their right hands to accommodate almost without thinking. If you are a left-handed woman, simply extend your hand, palm up; the person taking yours will automatically turn his wrist inward and hold your four fingers under his thumb. The

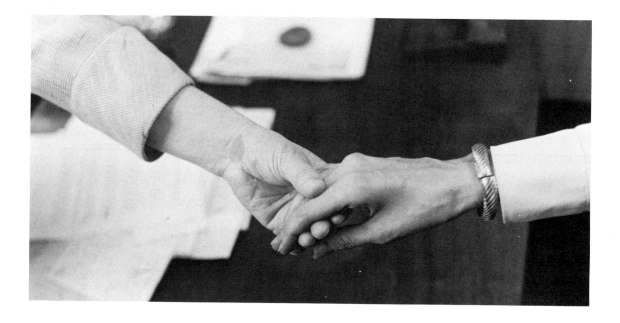

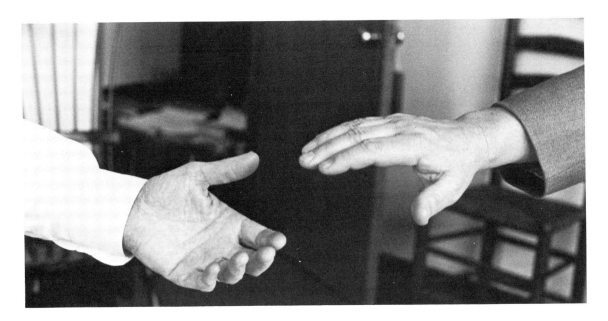

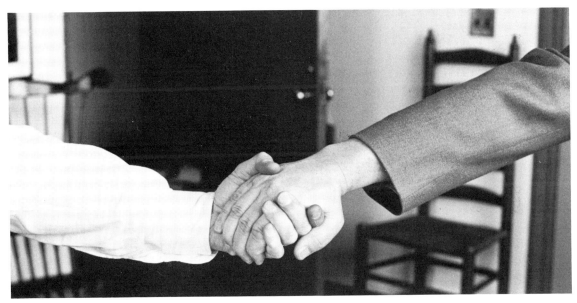

left-handed male will turn his palm outward and grasp his visitor's palm.

A man can help a woman into her coat by holding it with his forearm straddled across the inside neck and shoulder portion of the coat; that is, he can hold one sleeve under his elbow, gripping it to his chest, and insert his hand into the second shoulder to hold the coat secure. In this way the elbow takes the place of the second hand.

A one-handed woman getting into a coat

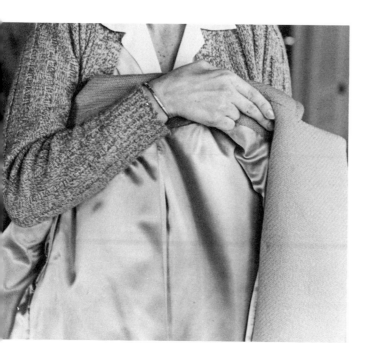
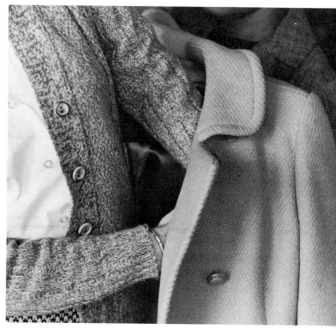

that is held for her should place her non-functioning arm into the sleeve first with the assistance of the good arm before putting her good arm through (see chapter 2, Dressing and Grooming).

The recent one-handed male dining out with a date can handle most cuts of meat on the menu (see chapter 11, Dining Out). If it is a first date for the one-handed girl or woman, she would order the easier-cutting meats mentioned in chapter 11. Sometimes a new escort or a friend or relative may ask if he can cut the meat if it appears difficult to handle. Agree to this with thanks. Chances are he will reach over and carve it in mere seconds.

When you attend a party where drinks are served, you will do well to position yourself at or near a table, mantel or bookcase, on which you can put down your drink for these situa-

tions which usually arise: introductions are being made and you want to shake hands; you want to light a cigarette or offer a light or cigarette to someone else; you want to help yourself to the hors d'oeuvres tray being passed around.

When entertaining at home you will find a serving cart almost as helpful as a servant (see chapter 7, In the Kitchen). It can double as a portable bar and will hold hors d'oeuvres, glasses, and all the paraphernalia necessary for entertaining. What a breeze for the host or hostess to wheel in canapés or coffee for a number of friends. One-handers who prefer to serve their guests from a tray should shop for medium-sized, lightweight trays made of aluminum or plastic. Larger trays must have an over-the-top handle to be lifted easily. (For tips on carrying a tray of food see chapter 11, Dining Out.)

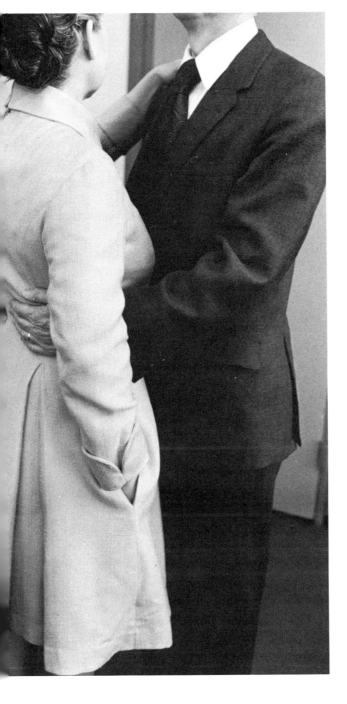

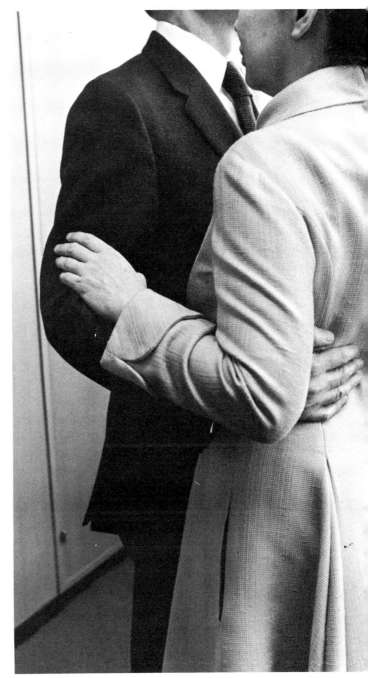

One-handers can enjoy dancing to their heart's content. Twist-style dancing, which requires a constant bobbing motion, will be comfortable for those who have no second arm, or who have an artificial arm that can be locked into position. Generally, fast dancing will not be comfortable for those with flail, or loosely hanging arms, but if you attempt this kind of dancing, one obvious help is a secure pocket in which to slip the hand. An arm sling (see chapter 17, Sports) made from a dressy material for girls or a solid, dark color for men is another aid. Of course a sling is not needed for ordinary dancing.

For ballroom dancing we have to consider the separate dance positions of men and women who have either a good right or a good left hand.

Left-handed women and girls take the normal position of placing their left arm at their partner's right shoulder. If you have a nonfunctioning right arm, you can place it in the pocket of your dress. Or your partner can hold your nonfunctioning right hand in his hand in the natural position. Or finally, assuming that your partner is someone you are very comfortable with, you can engage his help in clasping both your hands at the back of his neck—that is, your left hand will hold the right one in place there. (This is a comfortable dancing position and of course works smoothest between couples who know one another well.)

The female right-hander can either place her left hand into a dress pocket or position it on the right forearm of her partner, with the fingers resting against his upper arm in a quite natural dance position. It is true that this left arm, whether it is paralyzed or artificial, may have to be steadied now and again, especially if the dance tempo increases, but this position is the most comfortable and natural looking. And a right-hander too can clasp both hands behind her partner's neck, as described above for left-handers.

A left-handed man who has an artificial right arm can assume a natural dance position if he first locks the prosthesis into a right angle at the elbow. His partner can then posi-

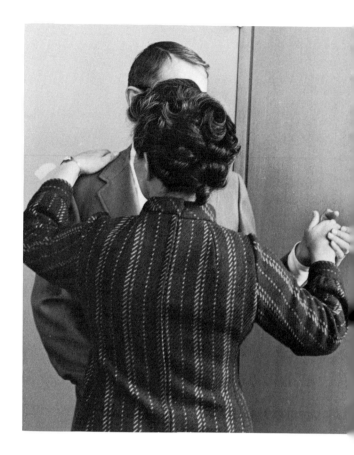

tion herself in the semicircle thus formed. Or he can place his right hand or jacket sleeve (in the absence of an arm) into his jacket pocket while his partner brings her hand to bear lightly on his right shoulder. He of course leads with his left in this position. This may take some getting used to, especially if the right arm was previously the dominant one. With practice his partner should be able to follow without having to be guided by arm pressure at her back. Another comfortable

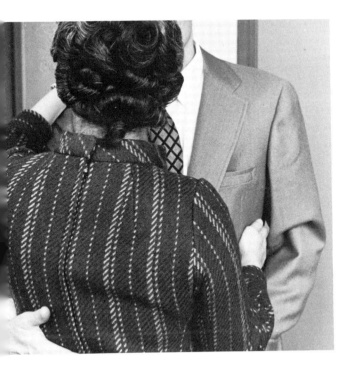

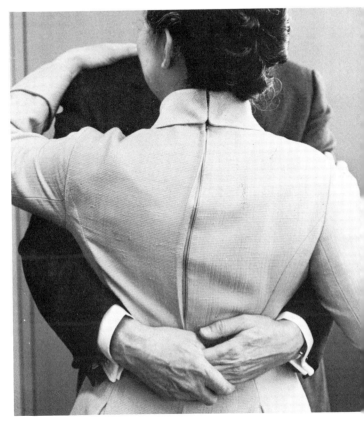

position for the man is to clasp both arms around his partner's waist, enlisting her assistance as needed. Again, this position works smoothest between couples who are completely at ease with each other.

A male right-hander can take the standard position, placing his arm at the woman's waist or back. The left hand or jacket sleeve can be inserted into his jacket pocket. His partner brings her right arm to bear lightly at his left shoulder or his left side. This position

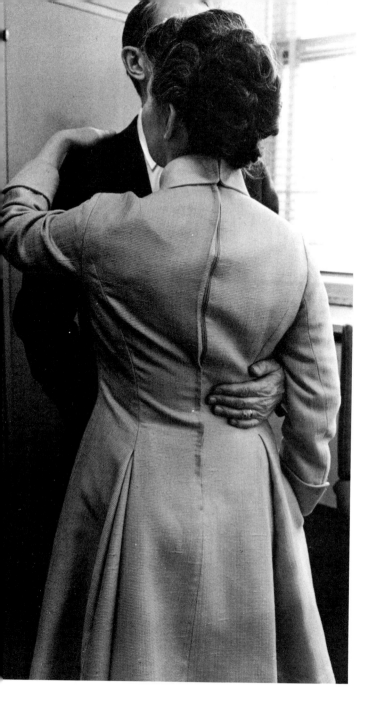

is quite natural looking. If the male right-hander has an artificial left arm which is flexible, his partner may choose to hold this hand in the standard dance position. Or, with his partner's aid he can clasp both hands around her waist, as described above for left-handed men.

When both dancing partners are one-handed, the most comfortable combination that works for appearance and ease of movement calls for both the man and woman to be either right- or left-handed. This combination joins the couple diagonally instead of laterally, which lends a more natural sway and grace to the dance steps.

How does one applaud with one hand? —we do it from the lap. Be seated then place your other or artificial hand palm down on the thigh corresponding to it and strike the back of this hand gently with your good one in the usual clapping manner. If you do not have a second arm, it is perfectly natural to clap on the thigh that corresponds to your good arm. If the audience should rise and applaud you would stand but not attempt clapping.

16

RECREATION

The more activities you engage in, the greater the chance that you will lose self-consciousness and enjoy yourself thoroughly. This holds true for everyone. Recent one-handers should continue with the hobbies that formerly gave them the greatest pleasure, which may be anything from sculpturing or woodcarving to furniture refinishing. If you like it well enough, there is no hobby your one-handedness will prevent you from enjoying.

To play card games, you can begin by using a card shuffler and card holder, but these are not essential to your playing. You will soon be able to shuffle and hold cards without these aids. Shuffling cards can take place either in your lap or, when you have achieved better finger dexterity, right in your hand. Here is how you can shuffle from your lap: cross your legs and prop the deck vertically against your thigh; grasp one half of the deck

and work this into the remaining cards still resting at your thigh. Repeat this several times and your cards are as shuffled as they need be.

The hand technique will take longer but it is not too difficult to master. It works best with a deck that is not too slick or new. Grasp the full deck by the longer edge at a right angle to the table (on which it rests). Your thumb and little finger are positioned one at each end of the shorter sides of the deck. If you raise your hand slightly while gripping the short edges, the center cards will remain intact, supported at your lower palm; you will have brought up the cards from the front and back of the deck. Hold this half securely in your index fingers and allow the second half to rest against your lower palm. You now drop the cards you are holding, interlacing them down among the second half (both halves are in their original positions) and

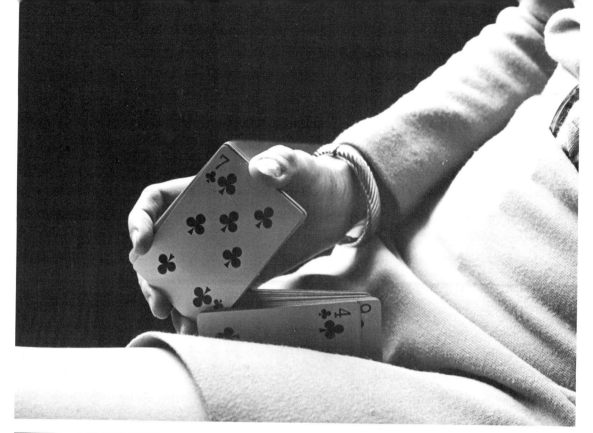

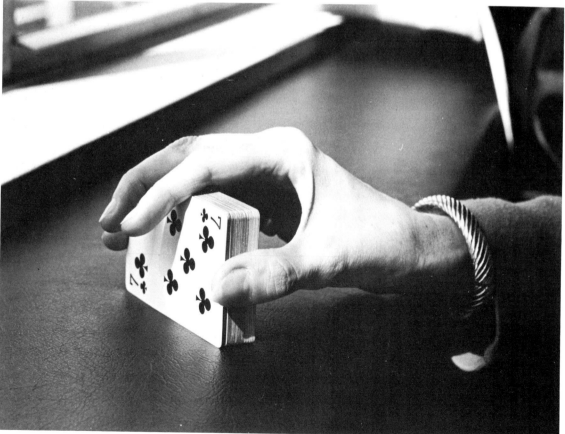

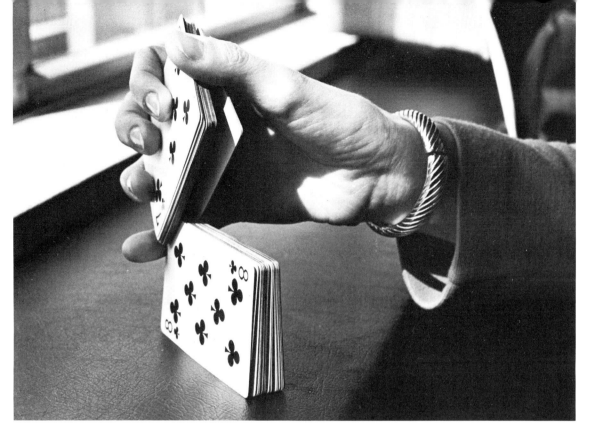

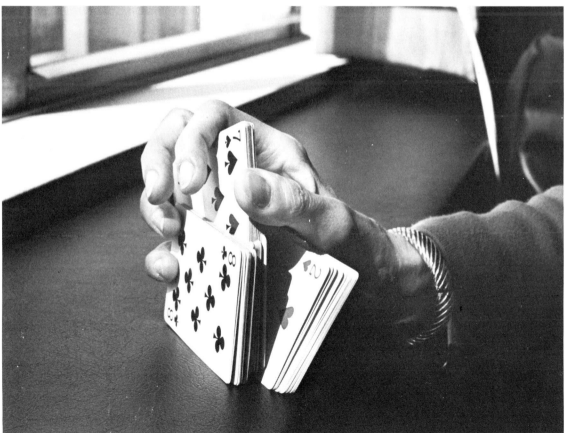

shuffling has taken place. Repeat this several times and you have done as well as if you had shuffled the cards with two hands.

Dealing with one hand is easy, especially if you deal half the deck at a time—with either the full deck or a half, simply slide each card from the top with the aid of your thumb.

If you want to use a card holder, fine. But if you play at a table you can either spread your cards in your lap, or if you have your other or an artificial hand, rest it on your lap and secure the cards between the thumb and index finger of this hand. This works fairly well, particularly if you hold a small hand of cards. If you do not have your second arm and you play cards in an open circle, you might do better to use a card holder.

One-handers who are musically inclined can play a number of instruments with fair proficiency, namely the piano, organ, a small accordian, the tuba, xylophone (vibes), a drum that has a foot hammer, and others. Your determination combined with a musical bent will see you through. You simply must be ready to devise ways to express your talent.

Composers such as Bach, Scriabin, Ravel, and Debussy have written piano music to be played with one hand. These are beautiful pieces of music, full and complete in sound, which can be mastered with practice by the person who has attained proficiency at the piano prior to becoming one-handed.

One-handers without previous musical training who are nevertheless determined to play will derive satisfaction from playing the treble staff in the original versions of music, omitting the base notes. Frequently simplified arrangements of the most popular current and classical music are available. In fact, re-cent one-handers without previous knowledge of the piano should begin their serious playing with simplified arrangements. Recent or long-term one-handers with a knowledge of harmony and of the piano will enjoy creating their own simplified versions of original music.

There is a technique for one-handers who want to play the melody and also include a few base notes or chords. This works easiest for music in slow tempo or on such pieces as the "Blue Danube Waltz," where a single base chord struck intermittently and sustained by the foot pedal provides enough base to complete the sound. This technique, which is easier for right-handers than left-handers, works as follows: move your hand to the left keyboard to strike the base chord; simultaneously press the hold foot pedal; return to the treble to strike the notes or chords of the melody. The sound of the music is complete and gives the effect of the instrument being played with both hands. The right hand must move quickly from the base to the treble chords but is assisted here by the holding pedal. This will take some practice in the beginning but becomes a satisfying variation of piano playing.

Left-handers will be more comfortable at the bass keyboard than at the treble keys. The technique for left-handers is essentially the same, although they will give more play to the bass, of course, and strike notes of the melody rather than chords. Left-handers can sing the melody while they are learning the bass chords.

Organ playing seems a natural for one-handers, because one or both feet can pump the bass chords.

114

A small accordian may be played by one-handers in this way: be seated and rest the base of the instrument on your knees. You will have first tied a piece of chord firmly to the handle strap of the bellows, leaving sufficient slack to reach the floor, and looped the other end into a noose through which you place the toe of your shoe. Your foot takes the place of your second arm, pulling the bellows open while your hand operates the keyboard. To deflate the bellows, position the accordian against the knee opposite to your good hand. Raise your knee slightly to meet it, at the same time applying firm pressure to the notes on the keyboard. The combined pressure from your hand and knee "sandwiches" the bellows for closing. This technique really does work, although it may seem strange in the reading. Practice is what it takes. Of course, playing this way may appeal more to the amateur than the advanced, former two-handed player, who might be dismayed at the absence of bass chords. Doubtless, a way could be devised to play bass chords if one were to think about it hard enough.

Small wind instruments with few finger valves, such as the piccolo, may be played with one hand. For long practice sessions the player can ease the tension of holding the instrument upright by sitting down and supporting the head of the instrument on a stand that is about level with the shoulders.

The harmonica is perhaps the easiest instrument for one-handers to play. To achieve the "trilling" effect, grip the harmonica between your teeth and vibrate the sound waves with your good hand. Here your teeth take over the function of a second hand. One-handers who are musically inclined but who have refrained from learning to play an instrument might well begin with the harmonica.

Whether you are left- or right-handed, you should be capable of driving a car competently and safely. One-handed drivers should be guided in the required equipment for their vehicles by individual state laws. Most states require the use of automatic transmission by one-handed drivers. A wheel spinner, which is a small knob attached by a screw to the steering wheel, that allows for easy turning of the wheel, as needed when parking for instance, is a device commonly required. Some states require a foot emergency brake and others may require power steering. The wheel spinner is probably the only special equipment required for one-handers, however. (Right-handers attach the spinner to the right of center of the wheel, and left-handers to the left.) Power steering is a boon to one-handers and strongly recommended for the exceptional comfort it provides. When signaling direction, move your wrist to the center knob of the wheel to steady it and flick the directional on with your thumb and first two fingers.

Right-handed drivers who are short or have small frames may have difficulty reaching for toll baskets and toll collectors from the driving side. One way to solve this problem is to keep handy a small straw basket which has a handle and simply "pass the basket" through the window to the collector. This may startle the collector but it will certainly reduce the strain on you. Right-handed drivers may also prefer push-button windows, particularly for ease and comfort in long-

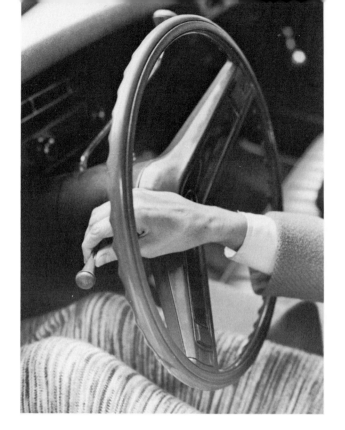

distance tollroad driving. And all one-handed drivers would do well to keep a supply of coins within hand's reach and so have the exact toll ready when needed.

Taking photographs does not require the use of two hands, although you may find it difficult in the beginning to hold the camera steady and simultaneously click the shutter. A lightweight camera will serve you best. Heavy professional cameras need the support of a tripod. Loading the camera is simple if it is one that takes a film cartridge.

What applies to two-handers applies to one-handers as well: the more recreational activities and hobbies one can cultivate, the greater will be the rewards and gratifications in one's life and the less the likelihood of withdrawing into a self-imposed isolation.

17

SPORTS

There are many sports which you can enjoy and participate in very ably. Bowling, fencing, and pitching ball seem to have been made for one-handers. Badminton, tennis, ice skating and roller skating—even skiing and other fast sports—can be mastered by the one-handed person, whether he is an amputee or has a paralysis or a birth defect. And no one needs two hands to hike or jog.

One suggestion that might be helpful to the sports-minded person with a paralysis who wants to engage in the faster sports just mentioned is the use of an arm sling. When one has a flail or loosely hanging arm, it is more comfortable dashing around a court, running the mile, or skating, etc., if the arm is supported at shoulder, elbow, and wrist with a simple arm sling. To make the sling, take a large square of cotton or any suitable fabric and fold it diagonally into a triangle. Knot the two ends together beforehand, then slip this over the neck. Place your arm into the fold

and secure the flap of the sling around your elbow. Safety-pin it here and at your wrist (pinning it to your shirt front) and you're all set. This will give you great freedom to run and play hard for long periods of time.

Slings need not be "institution white" either, though cotton gives firmer support than the synthetics of rayon or nylon; they can be color coordinated to match any outfit. We have seen slings of black satin and ones with splashy flowers, but, to repeat, arm slings are not needed except in cases of a flail arm or a loosely connected shoulder joint.

One-handers can serve in badminton by holding the racket and shuttlecock together in the hand. First grasp the racket in the usual manner, then pick up the bird between your thumb and index finger. This is your serving position. Now swing your arm down and on the upswing toss the bird straight up over your head, swinging your racket back to strike

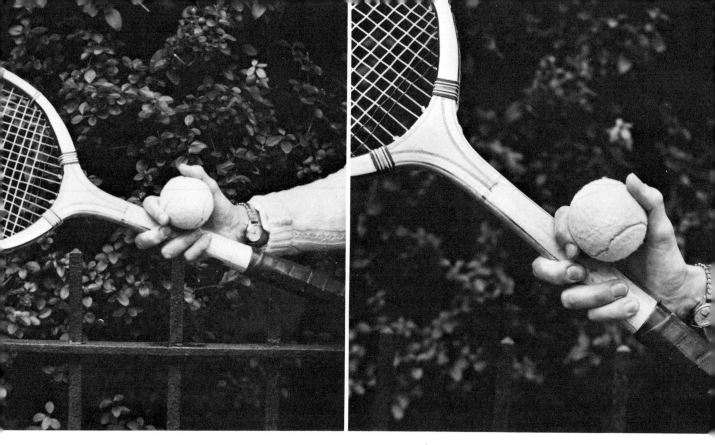

If your hand is not large, it is easier to grip the upper end of the racket handle while holding the ball. Steady the end of the racket handle against your waist. As soon as you have released the ball, shift your hand quickly to the leather-covered grip area in the approved handshake position ready to swing. With practice you will be able to hit the ball at the right moment of its rise from the bounce.

it. A tennis serve can be accomplished in the same way, or you may first bounce the ball and strike it on the ascent. If you have a small hand, you may prefer to do this. With a little practice you should be able to serve well.

Anyone who has formerly skied with two hands should not have much difficulty adjusting to one-hand skiing. You may prefer to use a pole or you may find that it interferes with your balance. Try both methods and decide which is better for you. Here again, one-handers with a paralysis may benefit from an arm sling.

Those one-handers who have otherwise normal muscle strength, such as amputees or accident victims but have never skied before, can usually ski in safety. But skiing is one of the sports that a person with general muscle weakness might well avoid, because he stands a greater chance of being injured. (However, if this person is determined to ski, he should go ahead and try it. Most of us know instinctively how much we can take and when to stop.) As a point of information for would-be skiers who live in the north-eastern section of the country, as of this writing there is a group in Vermont that specializes in teaching persons with physical impairments of all kinds how to ski.

One-handers can learn to swim fairly easily. Usually, children learn more quickly and with less fear, but with proper instruction adult one-handers also can learn to swim. To the recent one-hander, child or adult, who formerly swam with both arms, adjustment to one-arm swimming should be minor, because the technique has already been learned. Even beginning swimmers, children or adults, can adapt to one-arm swimming. The backcrawl and crawl are adaptable to one-handers and look much the same, although swimming speed is reduced. The sidestroke is almost identical. Keep in mind that your legs and feet do much of the work in swimming, assuming both are fairly strong. The leg opposite to your good arm will compensate by keeping you on a straight course.

Without breaking these strokes down in great detail, here are the basic techniques: for the backcrawl, lie on the water with your spine pushed slightly upward, legs together stretched straight out; the position is that of floating. Now, while your legs rhythmically scissor-cut the water, raise your arm (cup the fingers) out of the water above your head, brushing past your ear. Continue the circle backward down toward your thigh, making a complete revolution through the water. This is enough to propel you; you're off and swimming.

A modified sidestroke is easiest to do because there is little stretching and pulling. Lie on the side of your nonfunctioning arm, scissor-cutting the water with your legs. Now, with your fingers cupped, "paw" the water, making circular motions covering an area from about chest to hip. This stroke will take you the farthest distance with the most ease.

For the crawl, float face down, your good arm outstretched, legs together, with head held up or resting on one side in the water. If you are a right-handed swimmer, your head faces your left shoulder; if you are a left-handed swimmer your head faces the right shoulder. Your good arm is extended above your head, knees are slightly bent, toes inward, and you use the scissor kick. It should go like this: employing the scissor kick, propel your body forward. Inhale, bring your arm, fingers cupped, from the outstretched position straight down through the water; pivot your head through the water halfway toward the shoulder of your good arm, which is now rising from the water, and exhale in the water by blowing the air out through your nose. Your mouth, of course, is closed. As your arm comes forward for the next stroke, turn your face, still in the water, toward your other shoulder. You should be back in the position from which you started. You have completed the full stroke and are ready to inhale and repeat. The synchronization of the arm and head movements becomes automatic after a while. You can practice this at home lying across a twin-size bed so that your arms and legs are free to move.

If you prefer to swim with your head above the water, you have just to synchronize your arm and leg movements.

If you have your other arm, unless it is immobile due to a surgical operation, you can use it to advantage in diving. Try it this way: stand at the edge of the pool or diving board (or dock, boat, etc.) with toes gripping this surface. Take the fingers of your nonfunctioning hand in your good one, and raise both arms to shoulder height. Lower your head between the arch formed by your arms and plunge off, chin down, by pushing from the pool's edge with your feet. (Beginners can practice diving from a kneeling position on the board or at poolside to perfect the technique and to lessen the fear of the longer fall.) Eventually you will be able to dive comfortably from boards of varying heights in just this way, and it will look almost as if you were diving with two good arms. If you have the stump of your upper forearm the muscles there and in your shoulder will assist your dive and help your balance, even though you hit the water with one arm. Poise your body in the same position described above, and off you go.

Can the one-handed person safely ride a bicycle? Certainly—if one learned to ride as a child, either one-handed or with both hands. Once balance has been mastered, biking with one arm is effortless. Adult one-handers who never learned to ride as children but who otherwise have good muscles and coordination will gain their balance quickly and perhaps even ride on the second try.

The difficulty for children or adult one-handers who, with generally weakened musculature (the aftermath of polio, for example), would nevertheless like to take up bicycling is that the bike may be heavy to handle.

Pedaling and maintaining balance may therefore not be easy. A few suggestions which may help are to use a lightweight bicycle, to experiment with training wheels, and to raise the handlebars slightly higher than standard for more sitting comfort. Above all, strong motivation and practice are needed for such one-handers to master this skill. We have all seen two-handers glide along holding on with one hand and even with no hands, so we know it can be done. For those adults who may not want to put in the time and effort that is required to master the bicycle, the adult tricycle provides a very comfortable ride. Not all rental outlets keep them in stock and fewer of them are manufactured than bicycles of course, but they are available.

Fishing for small catch with one hand can be effected comfortably with a little practice. In a sitting position, grip the rod handle between your knees to steady it before you reel in the catch with your hand. The rod will wobble at first until your knees are accustomed to holding it steady in coordination with the winding of the reel. To affix bait easily, secure the hook under your foot and work the bait over the hook's point. Stringing the pole or unhooking the fish can best be managed by the one-hander with the pole lying on the ground. Your knees and good arm can then steady the pole or subdue a wriggling three-pounder.

ONE LAST WORD

It was the author's intention to include most of the major normal life activities the one-handed person would encounter. Because of the many variables in individual life styles, it was neither possible nor advisable to cover all situations that might arise. Rather, we have sought to motivate the reader to seek his own adaptations and original techniques, meeting new situations as they arise. Thus, many one-handed persons may eventually develop methods that will operate even better for them than the ones detailed in this handbook. All are encouraged to adopt any procedure that simplifies living for them.

INDEX